PRIMARY CARE FOR PHYSICIAN ASSISTANTS

PreTest® Self-Assessment and Review

NOTICE

PRIMARY CARE FOR PHYSICIAN ASSISTANTS

PreTest® Self-Assessment and Review

Editor

Rodney L. Moser, PA-C, PhD

Assistant Professor
Director of Clinical Education
Physician Assistant Program
Central Michigan University
Mount Pleasant, Michigan

McGraw-Hill

Health Professions Division

PreTest® Series

New York   St. Louis   San Francisco   Auckland   Bogotá   Caracas   Lisbon   London
Madrid   Mexico City   Milan   Montreal   New Delhi   San Juan   Singapore   Sydney   Tokyo   Toronto

McGraw-Hill

*A Division of The **McGraw·Hill** Companies*

Primary Care for Physician Assistants
PreTest® Self-Assessment and Review

2 3 4 5 6 7 8 9 0   MALMAL   9 9 8

ISBN 0-07-052406-8

This book was set in Times Roman by V&M Graphics, Inc.
The editors were John J. Dolan, Lucinda C. Bauer, and Lester A. Sheinis.
The production supervisor was Helene G. Landers.
The text designer was Robert Freese.
The cover designer was Joan O'Connor.
Malloy Lithographing, Inc., was printer and binder.

This book is printed on acid-free paper.

CONTENTS

Contributors   *vii*
Preface   *xi*
Test Wiseness   *xiii*
  Steven H. Stumpf
Stress Management for Test Takers   *xv*
  Jack Liskin

Section 1. Cardiovascular   1
        Questions   3
        Answers, Explanations, and References   7

Section 2. Dermatology   13
        Questions   15
        Answers, Explanations, and References   21

Section 3. Ear, Nose, and Throat   31
        Questions   33
        Answers, Explanations, and References   36

Section 4. Emergency Medicine   39
        Questions   41
        Answers, Explanations, and References   44

Section 5. Endocrinology   49
        Questions   51
        Answers, Explanations, and References   56

Section 6. Gastroenterology   63
        Questions   65
        Answers, Explanations, and References   73

Section 7. Hematology   83
      Questions   85
      Answers, Explanations, and References   87

Section 8. Infectious Disease   91
      Questions   93
      Answers, Explanations, and References   100

Section 9. Musculoskeletal   109
      Questions   111
      Answers, Explanations, and References   116

Section 10. Neurology   123
      Questions   125
      Answers, Explanations, and References   128

Section 11. Obstetrics/Gynecology   133
      Questions   135
      Answers, Explanations, and References   140

Section 12. Oncology   147
      Questions   149
      Answers, Explanations, and References   153

Section 13. Ophthalmology   159
      Questions   161
      Answers, Explanations, and References   164

Section 14. Pediatrics   167
      Questions   169
      Answers, Explanations, and References   174

Section 15. Psychiatry   179
      Questions   181
      Answers, Explanations, and References   184

Section 16. Respiratory   189
      Questions   191
      Answers, Explanations, and References   194

Section 17. Urology   199
      Questions   201
      Answers, Explanations, and References   204

Bibliography   *207*

CONTRIBUTORS

David P. Asprey, MA, PA-C
Interim Program Director
University of Iowa PA Program
Physician Assistant
Division of Pediatric Cardiology
University of Iowa Hospitals and Clinics
Iowa City, Iowa

Martin Beatty, BS, PA-S, HMCS(SS), USN(ret)
Physician Assistant Program
Central Michigan University
Mount Pleasant, Michigan

Barry A. Cassidy, PhD, PA-C
Associate Professor and Associate Director
Physician Assistant Program
Midwestern University—Glendale Campus
Glendale, Arizona

Stephen M. Cohen, MS, PA-C
Academic Director and Assistant Professor
Physician Assistant Program
Nova Southeastern University
Fort Lauderdale, Florida

Jean M. Covino, PA-C, MPA
Adjunct Associate Professor
Physician Assistant Program
University of Medicine and Dentistry of New Jersey
Piscataway, New Jersey

Rick Davis, PA-C
Senior Physician Assistant
Division of Gastroenterology, Hepatology, and Nutrition
University of Florida
Gainesville, Florida

Meredith Davison, PhD
Associate Professor and Master's Education Director
Physician Assistant Program
Midwestern University
Downers Grove, Illinois

JoAnn Deasy, PA-C, MPH
Director
Physician Assistant Program
Catholic Medical Center of Brooklyn and Queens, Inc.
Jamaica, New York

Richard Dehn, MPA, PA-C
Assistant Director
Physician Assistant Program
University of Iowa
Iowa City, Iowa

Morton A. Diamond, MD, FACP, FACC, FAHA
Professor and Medical Director
Physician Assistant Program
Nova Southeastern University
Fort Lauderdale, Florida

Michelle DiBaise, MPAS, PA-C
Physician Assistant and Clinical Research Coordinator
Division of Dermatology
University of Nebraska Medical Center
Omaha, Nebraska

Kathleen J. Dobbs, PA-C, MS
Faculty Specialist
College of Osteopathic Medicine
Michigan State University
East Lansing, Michigan

Timothy C. Evans, MD, PhD
Acting Assistant Professor
School of Medicine
University of Washington
Seattle, Washington

William H. Fenn, PhD, PA-C
Associate Professor
Physician Assistant Department
Western Michigan University
Kalamazoo, Michigan

Dana M. Gallagher, PA-C, MPH
Monterey, California

Noel J. Genova, MA, PA-C
Staff Physician Assistant
Mercy Family Practice
Portland, Maine
Adjunct Faculty, Research Advisor
Physician Assistant Program
University of New England
Biddeford, Maine

Anita D. Glicken, MSW
Associate Professor and Psychosocial Coordinator
Child Health Association Physician Assistant Program
University of Colorado Health Science Center
Denver, Colorado

Meredith Hansen, MPH, PA-C
Associate Director and Assistant Professor
Physician Assistant Studies Program
The University of Texas Health Science
*   Center–San Antonio*
San Antonio, Texas

Anne P. Heinly, PA-C, MMS, MPS
Major, USAF, BSC
Program Supervisor, Phase II, Offut Air Force Base
Interservice Physician Assistant Program–USAF Branch
Associate Professor of Medicine
University of Nebraska Medical Center
Omaha, Nebraska

Janice Herbert-Carter, MD, MGA, FACP
Morehouse School of Medicine
Department of Medical Education
Atlanta, Georgia

Laura Hess, MSN, ANP
Adult Nurse Practitioner
Sutter Medical Group
Sacramento, California

Katherine D. Hocum, BS, PA-C
Physician Assistant
Federal Medical Center
Rochester, Minnesota

Pat C.H. Jan, MS, PA-C
Adjunct Faculty
Physician Assistant Program
Midwestern University
Downers Grove, Illinois
Surgical Physician Assistant and
*   PA Educational Coordinator*
Thorek Hospital and Medical Center
Chicago, Illinois

Patricia Kelly, MHS, PA-C
Assistant Professor
Director of Didactic Education
Physician Assistant Program
Central Michigan University
Mount Pleasant, Michigan

Nadine Kroenke, PA-C
Staff Physician Assistant
Emergency Medicine Specialists
Milwaukee, Wisconsin

Jack Liskin, MA, PA-C
Assistant Professor of Clinical Family Medicine
School of Medicine
University of Southern California
Los Angeles, California

Dennis Loudenback, MHS, PA-C
Vascular Surgery
Seattle, Washington

Sandra J. Martin, DPM, PA
Department of Orthopaedics
UC Davis Medical Group
University of California, Davis Medical Center
Sacramento, California

Marquitha S. Mayfield, MEd, PA-C
Assistant Professor and Academic Coordinator
Physician Assistant Program
Emory University School of Medicine
Atlanta, Georgia

Joe R. Monroe, PA-C, MPAS
Founder
Society of Dermatology Physician Assistants, Inc.
Vancouver, Washington

Rodney L. Moser, PA-C, PhD
Assistant Professor
Director of Clinical Education
Physician Assistant Program
Central Michigan University
Mount Pleasant, Michigan

William A. Mosier, MPAS, EdD, PA-C
Director of Research
Center for the Study of Child Development
San Antonio, Texas

Amelia Naccarto-Coleman, PA-C, MAS
Instructor
Physician Assistant Education
Primary Care Physician Assistant Program
College of Allied Health Professions
Western University of Health Sciences
Pomona, California

Karen A. Newell, PA-C
Academic Coordinator
Physician Assistant Program
Emory University School of Medicine
Atlanta, Georgia

Claire Babcock O'Connell, MPH, PA-C
Physician Assistant Program
University of Medicine and Dentistry of New Jersey
Piscataway, New Jersey

Maureen MacLeod O'Hara, PA-C
Geriatric Physician Assistant
HealthCare Partners Medical Group
Los Angeles, California

Patti Pagels, PA-C
Instructor
Department of Family Medicine
Health Science Center
University of North Texas
Fort Worth, Texas

Kimberly Brown Paterson, MS, RD, PA-C
Emergency Medicine Physician Assistant
Eastern Carolina Emergency Physicians
Wilmington, North Carolina

Jill Reichman, MPH, PA-C
Assistant Director and Associate Professor
Rutgers University Physician Assistant Program
University of Medicine and Dentistry of New Jersey
Piscataway, New Jersey

Ralph Rice, PA-C
Clinical Assistant Professor
Physician Assistant Program
University of Florida
Gainesville, Florida

Allan R. Riggs, MS, PA-C
Assistant Professor
Physician Assistant Program
Central Michigan University
Mount Pleasant, Michigan

Barbara L. Sauls, MS, PA-C
Clinical Director
Physician Assistant Program
King's College
Wilkes-Barre, Pennsylvania

Thomas J. Schymanski, PA-C
Captain
U.S. Army
Physician Assistant
Family Health Center of Fort Belvoir
DeWitt Army Community Hospital
Fort Belvoir, Virginia

Pamela Moyers Scott, PA-C
Rainelle Medical Center
Rainelle, West Virginia

Donald J. Sefcik, DO, MS, RPh
Medical Director
Associate Professor
Physician Assistant Program
Midwestern University
Downers Grove, Illinois

Freddi Segal-Gidan, PA, PhD
Department of Neurological Sciences and Gerontology
Alzheimer's Disease Diagnostic and Treatment Center
Rancho Los Amigos Medical Center
Downey, California

Howell J. Smith III, MMS, PA-C
Associate Director and Assistant Professor
Physician Assistant Program
Nova Southeastern University
Fort Lauderdale, Florida

Jeffery R. Smith, PA-C
Family Practice and Sports Medicine
Rockwood Clinic, PS
Spokane, Washington

Christopher C. Stephanoff, MA, PA-C
Academic Coordinator
Physician Assistant Program
Medical University of South Carolina
Charleston, South Carolina

Don St. John, MA, PA
Physician Assistant
Adult Outpatient Psychiatry
University of Iowa Hospitals and Clinics
Iowa City, Iowa

Steven H. Stumpf, EdD
Director of Education, Research, and Evaluation
Department of Family Medicine
University of Southern California School of Medicine
Los Angeles, California

Randy Trudeau, PA-C
Physician Assistant
St. Ignatius, Montana

Peggy Valentine, EdD, PA-C
Associate Professor
Physician Assistant Department
Director of National AIDS Minority Information
  and Education Program
Howard University
Washington, DC

Wayne J. van Deusen, PA-C
Pediatric Provider
Berkeley Primary Care Access Clinic
Berkeley, California

Suzanne Warnimont, PA-C, MPH
Director and Chairperson
Physician Assistant Program
University of Detroit Mercy
Detroit, Michigan

Andrea G. Weiss, PA-C
Physician Assistant
Sacramento, California

David Zinsmeister, MMS, PA-C
Director
Physician Assistant Program
Assistant Dean
College of Allied Health
Nova Southeastern University
Fort Lauderdale, Florida

PREFACE

This PreTest® Self-Assessment and Review, which accompanies *Primary Care for Physician Assistants,* has been designed to prepare students for the Physician Assistant National Certification Examination (PANCE). The nearly 700 questions cover the clinical topics in *Primary Care for Physician Assistants.* Practicing PAs looking to recertify or needing a review book will also benefit from this text.

With up-to-date references, the book can be used as a quick study guide. All of the questions follow the National Commission on Certification of Physician Assistants (NCCPA) guidelines.

This is the second book in our *Primary Care for Physician Assistants* series. A Companion Handbook will complete the package.

TEST WISENESS

Steven H. Stumpf

It is possible to improve your chances of scoring well by using test-wiseness strategies. This chapter reviews some of the most recent research on this broad topic and, hopefully, guides you toward the best and most successful strategies, which will increase your chances to do your absolute best.

What is test wiseness? It is the "capacity to utilize the characteristics and formats of a test and/or the test-taking situation to receive a high score."[1] In other words, it is the test taker's ability to use information other than specific knowledge—such as aspects of the test itself—to gain an advantage in identifying the correct response. There are two kinds of advantages available to the test taker: strategies not to lose points, and strategies to gain points.[2]

Not losing points is a matter of using commonsense techniques, such as the basic time management scheme.

Basic Time Management Scheme

1. Plan to make three runs through the exam.
2. Allow less than one minute per item for the initial run. Initially, answer only the items you are sure of; mark the ones you have an idea about; and leave unmarked the ones for which you haven't got a clue.
3. In your second run, answer the ones you marked using some of the deduction strategies discussed below, especially those for changing answers or inclinations.
4. In your third run, quickly check answers for mismarks on your answer sheet and take your best guesses on questions still left blank (see comments below).

Basic Deduction Strategies for Making the Best Choices

1. Find out as much as you can about the exam before taking the exam.
   - How many items will there be?
   - How much time is allowed for completing the exam?

   Divide the total items by the total time allowed to figure how much time is maximally available per item. Divide that in half and use it as your per item time limit for the first run through the exam.
   - Will there be a guessing adjustment built into the scoring?

In the past, the Physician Assistant National Certification Examination (PANCE) has only counted correct responses and has not adjusted scores for guessing. Therefore, a good, overall test-taking strategy should include tips on how to guess.

2. Eliminate choices that
   - are poorly written, e.g., they do not grammatically follow the stem;
   - are obviously incorrect or ridiculous;
   - do not belong in the same major group as the other choices;
   - are diametrically opposed to each other so that one, if not both, must be wrong;
   - are modified by *always, never,* and *none,* which tend to be associated with false items.

3. Highlight choices that are
   - repeated from other items (if a choice is used in two different items the two items may be linked in a way that illuminates correct or incorrect responses);
   - awkwardly written, e.g., use of double negatives may reveal an item writer struggling to construct a plausible false choice;
   - remarkably longer or shorter than the others;
   - more general or specific than the others;
   - grammatically consistent, e.g., the stem indicates the right answer begins with a consonant or a vowel;
   - modified by *usually, often,* and *many,* which tend to be associated with true items.

4. Increase the odds of guessing correctly to 50 percent by reducing your choices to no more than two for which you have no information.

Should You Change Your Answers?

Yes. Quite a bit of research has addressed this question.[3,4,5] Studies have demonstrated that when test takers change their answers they go from wrong to right more than half the time (some estimate the probability of changing a wrong answer to a right one is as high as 2:1). On the remaining occasions test takers are changing answers from wrong to wrong or from right to wrong. The benefits of changing answers on multiple-choice items can be increased if the test taker is also employing deduction strategies. Although changing answers is helpful to test takers of all ability levels, it is especially beneficial to those who tend to score highest.

Doesn't this contradict the basic time management strategy? Should you change answers from the first run through the exam? Probably not. The second run through the exam is when you want to change your mind regarding the answers about which you felt strongly, but were still less than certain.

What About Guessing?

In regard to the PANCE, it is clearly to the test taker's advantage to guess on unanswered items. This is because the test taker gets credit for every right answer and is not penalized by an adjustment formula for attempting extra items and guessing incorrectly on them. Some national exams such as the Scholastic Aptitude Test (SAT) adjust scores for guessing. Interestingly, it has been found that even when an adjustment is made for guessing "the more able examinees do tend to profit somewhat from guessing, and would therefore be disadvantaged by their reluctance to guess."[6]

Increase your odds at guessing by using deduction strategies to eliminate as many choices as you can. If you can increase your guessing odds to 50 percent (one of two), then you are in pretty good shape to take a blind stab.

Finally, review "Stress Management for Test Takers" on page xv and give it your best effort.

References

1. Millman J, Bishop CH, Ebel R: An analysis of test-wiseness. *Educ Psychol Meas* 25:707–726, 1965.
2. Towns MH, Robinson WR: Student use of test-wiseness strategies in solving multiple choice chemistry problems. *J Res Sci Teach* 30(7):709–722, 1993.
3. Schwarz SP, McMorris RF, DeMers LP: Reasons for changing answers: An evaluation using personal interviews. *J Educ Meas* 28(2):163–171, 1991.
4. Hanna GS: To change answers or not to change answers: That is the question. *Clear House* 62(9):414–416, 1989.
5. Casteel CA: Answer changing on multiple choice test items among eighth grade readers. *J Exp Educ* 59(4):300–309, 1991.
6. Angoff WH: Does guessing really help? *J Educ Meas* 26(4):323–336, 1989.

STRESS MANAGEMENT FOR TEST TAKERS

Jack Liskin

The "Yes" Set

You want to pass your exam. You will feel quite happy when you do. You may be afraid of not passing, but if you spend a moment you can recall that you have taken and passed many exams in your life. That means that you have recalled or figured out correctly many answers to many questions. You can pass this exam as you have so many others in your life. And, in fact, the large majority of people taking this particular exam do pass it. If you prepare yourself properly, your chances of passing will increase greatly.

Preparation and Practice

"How do you get to Carnegie Hall?" a tourist asked a native New Yorker. "Practice, practice," was the Manhattanite's advice. The best way to pass this exam is to learn or review the material and practice answering questions of the type you are likely to encounter, and to do that repeatedly over many weeks. That way, even if the stresses are great, your foundation will be strong and won't fall apart under the strain of the test situation. It may be fear that motivates you to prepare, or the drive to succeed, or something else. All of them are fine if they get you to spend the time you need to prepare; however, if you do your learning in a relaxed way it will be easier to recall the information in a relaxed way when you take the test.

Rehearsal

Mental rehearsal is slightly different from the preparation you do when you learn clinical content and practice the clinical skills needed for success. In athletics, a basketball player may rehearse by throwing an imaginary ball toward the hoop and seeing it swish through. So, too, you can rehearse by imagining yourself walking into the examination room, situating yourself comfortably, opening the exam booklet, reading the question calmly and thinking through the answer, letting go of that question and moving on to the next one at a steady pace, taking time for a relaxing breath or a stretch, and so on until you have moved through all of the answers and handed in the booklets. As the exam date gets closer, you can begin to rehearse in this way.

Expectations

Choose the best answer to the following question:

The least stressful expectation to have in taking an exam is to

(A) score 100 percent
(B) fail the exam
(C) do your best and pass
(D) have a terrible time and pass

If you answered anything other than C, reflect for a moment on how reasonable and helpful your expectations are. Often we have underlying expectations we don't realize are acting within us; ask yourself about your inner expectations. You may discover fear or something else unpleasant lurking somewhere in the shadows. If so, perform the most rational risk assessment you are capable of (you may need to ask a friend for a reality check here) and coach yourself in the direction of expectation C. That might mean repeating it like a mantra every morning and night until you believe it.

Mind Your Body/Help Your Mind

What do ballplayers and other performers say when interviewed after a particularly great performance? "I felt good" or "I was very comfortable out there." You also want to feel good and comfortable for your big "performance." That means spreading out your study and practice so that you don't have to lose sleep the week before the exam, and especially the night before. Eat before the exam, but nothing too heavy, and bring some energy snacks and drinks with you if they are allowed in the exam room. If you are on prescribed medications, make sure you take them before the exam or have them with you.

Find a spot in the room to sit comfortably, where you feel physically at ease, and where there are few distractions. If you need a cushion or lumbar support, bring one with you. Layer your clothing to suit different possible room temperatures.

Starting in the study and preparation phase, begin to practice simple techniques to relax if you don't already know or use them. That way you will be adept at using them when you need them most. If you understand relaxation as a kind of letting go, then you can recognize tension as a kind of holding on. But letting go does not mean that you cease to have control. For example, the watch you will bring into the exam room to help you pace yourself properly lets go of one moment in order to move on to the next one. If you find yourself holding on to one question too long, you can also let go and move on to the next one.

If you feel physical tension, find the part of your body that is tense and let it go. If you have trouble with that, tense that part purposely for an instant so you feel it better, then let it go.

If you tend to experience mental tension—that is, you find yourself straining to remember something—think about the last time you were able to recall something that was on the tip of your tongue. You probably either followed a line of associations until the right memory came in or you just let go and soon the information somehow bubbled up into your consciousness. During the exam, allow the information to emerge in these ways.

If you feel bound up or out of control or unfocused either physically or mentally, breathe as a relaxation tool. Since you breathe every four seconds or so, your breath is an ever-present therapeutic tool (remember too that it feeds your highly oxygen-dependent brain). Rather than force yourself to take in a deep breath, just let the old air out and feel the new air flow in. If you were to do that consciously one hundred times during the exam, you will use less than seven minutes of the time you have available.

While seated, you can take a moment periodically to stretch your arms and shoulders and chest (take a good breath while doing that), and when you stand or go for a break, take a moment to shake yourself out and relocate your center of gravity.

If your test stress runs deeper than what the foregoing tools can handle, consult a clinician or counselor for additional help. If you think you have a learning disability, get evaluated by qualified people. Otherwise, take a moment now to anticipate and enjoy the feeling of successfully passing your examination!

SECTION 1
CARDIOVASCULAR

1. CARDIOVASCULAR

QUESTIONS

DIRECTIONS: Each question below contains suggested responses. Choose the **one best** response to each question.

1-1. The earliest cardiac manifestation of hyperkalemia is

(A) absent P waves
(B) complete heart block
(C) depressed ST segment
(D) peaked T waves
(E) widened QRS

1-2. A 75-year-old female presents with acute onset of right arm weakness and clumsiness now resolving, as well as intermittent left arm and leg "heaviness" over several weeks. Her blood pressure is 125/70, pulse is 80 and irregular, and temperature is 37°C (98.6°F). The labs are unremarkable except for an INR of 1.3. Based on the presentation and findings reported here, the MOST likely cause of her symptoms is

(A) right carotid artery stenosis causing TIA
(B) left carotid artery stenosis causing TIA
(C) vertebrobasilar insufficiency from subclavian steal
(D) cardiogenic emboli from atrial fibrillation
(E) intracerebral hemorrhage causing elevated intracranial pressure

1-3. An 85-year-old male patient has a left carotid stenosis of 75 percent resulting in intracerebral "crossing over" and retrograde flow in the left ophthalmic artery. He has had no symptoms suggestive of stroke or TIA. Of the following options, which is the LEAST appropriate?

(A) referral to a neurologist for evaluation
(B) referral to a vascular surgeon for evaluation
(C) initiation of antiplatelet therapy
(D) repeat ultrasound at one year, or earlier if symptomatic
(E) obtain CT scan to rule out prior "silent" infarcts

1-4. Which of the following cardiac pathologies is the MOST common cause of stroke?

(A) recent myocardial infarction
(B) atrial fibrillation
(C) atrial/ventricular septal defects
(D) bacterial endocarditis
(E) mitral valve prolapse

1-5. Which of the following is NOT considered a risk factor for hemorrhagic stroke?

(A) atrial fibrillation
(B) hypertension
(C) cocaine/amphetamine use
(D) cerebral aneurysm
(E) warfarin (Coumadin) therapy

1-6. On routine physical examination a 55-year-old man with a history of a mild stable angina is found to have a bruit over the left neck that clearly does not emanate from the heart. After careful questioning by you it appears he has had no symptoms to suggest a previous stroke or TIA. The MOST appropriate step on your part would be to

(A) obtain a vascular surgery consultation in anticipation of surgery
(B) get a noncontrast head CT to rule out previous infarct
(C) obtain a neurology consultation to perform a more thorough exam
(D) reassure the patient, and encourage follow-up in 12 months
(E) get a Doppler ultrasound to determine the degree of stenosis

3

1-7. Abnormal lipid metabolism may be the result of

(A) genetics
(B) life-style risk factors
(C) diet
(D) medications
(E) all of the above

1-8. One of the least expensive and broadest spectrum medications to lower lipids is

(A) gemfibrozil
(B) fiber supplements
(C) niacin (nicotinic acid)
(D) aspirin
(E) pravastatin

1-9. Signs and symptoms of hyperlipidemia include

(A) xanthomas
(B) abdominal pain
(C) pale creamy blood samples
(D) yellow-orange discolorations in the creases of the palms of the hands
(E) all of the above

1-10. A 21-year-old man presents in the emergency department after using cocaine. Heart rhythm is sinus with rate of 140 per min. Blood pressure is 200/120. The patient is treated with propranolol. Fifteen minutes later the patient experiences severe chest pain and ECG demonstrates myocardial ischemia. Which is correct?

(A) the ischemia was precipitated by increased beta-sympathetic effect on coronary arteries
(B) the ischemia was precipitated by increased alpha-sympathetic and beta-sympathetic effect on coronary arteries
(C) the ischemia was precipitated by unopposed alpha-sympathetic effect on coronary arteries
(D) the ischemia was precipitated by acute thrombosis without sympathetic nervous system influence

1-11. A 69-year-old man presents to the emergency room with acute anterior chest pain and dyspnea. Puzzlement abounds in the emergency room as the staff struggles to differentiate acute myocardial infarction with pulmonary edema from pericarditis with tamponade. The physician assistant arrives and clarifies the problem by declaring

(A) an elevated central venous pressure (CVP) suggests acute pulmonary edema with acute myocardial infarction
(B) a paradoxical pulse suggests acute pulmonary edema
(C) an elevated CVP with paradoxical pulse suggests tamponade
(D) a low CVP with paradoxical pulse suggests tamponade

1-12. The risk of sudden death is increased in all the following EXCEPT

(A) smokers
(B) left ventricular hypertrophy
(C) paroxysmal atrial fibrillation
(D) left ventricular systolic dysfunction

1-13. A 72-year-old man with known angina pectoris presents in the emergency room with increased anginal frequency, now even awakening him from sleep. BP is 120/70; pulse 84 and regular. ECG shows ischemia of anterior wall of LV. Chest x-ray is normal. The physician assistant may properly use all the following medications in this patient EXCEPT

(A) aspirin
(B) beta blocker
(C) intravenous heparin
(D) angiotensin-converting enzyme (ACE) inhibitor

1-14. Risk factors for the development of coronary atherosclerosis include all the following EXCEPT

(A) postmenopausal state
(B) smoking
(C) hypertension
(D) elevated LDL cholesterol
(E) elevated HDL cholesterol

1-15. Stress echocardiograms demonstrate ischemia by

(A) inducing mitral regurgitation
(B) inducing transient ventricular wall motion abnormalities
(C) demonstrating permanent ventricular wall motion abnormalities
(D) inducing right atrial diastolic collapse

1-16. A 31-year-old woman presents with acute anterior chest pain worsening upon inspiration. History includes a 2-week history of diffuse joint pain as well as a burning sensation in the fingers when holding a package of frozen food. Patient is on no medication. Physical examination is consistent with acute pericarditis. Of the following one would expect

(A) patient to have positive smooth-muscle anti-body titer
(B) urine to show proteinuria and microscopic hematuria
(C) urine to show white blood cells, white blood cell casts, and urate crystals
(D) blood to reveal elevated hematocrit, elevated white blood count, and thrombocytopenia

1-17. In a patient who has chronic nonvalvular atrial fibrillation and who has sustained a stroke due to cardiac embolism, the preferred long-term therapy in preventing a recurrent stroke is

(A) aspirin
(B) ticlopidine
(C) warfarin
(D) liparin

1-18. Serum cholesterol may be divided into several subclasses. Elevations in which of the following total cholesterol subclasses should be aggressively treated to reduce risk for atherosclerosis?

(A) LDL-C and its subclasses
(B) HDL-C and its subclasses
(C) triglycerides and chylomicrons
(D) total cholesterol only

1-19. Acute cardiac or vascular ischemic events are usually associated with which ONE of the following pathological changes?

(A) vessel occlusion/obstruction by atherosclerotic plaque
(B) acute vasospasm and hypertension
(C) thrombosis formation at the site of a ruptured atherosclerotic plaque
(D) heavily calcified atherosclerotic plaque with significant vessel occlusion

1-20. Benefits of reducing serum lipid levels may include

(A) regression of atherosclerotic plaque
(B) primary prevention of atherosclerosis
(C) reduction of risk for cardiovascular disease
(D) normalization of cholesterol subclass production and utilization
(E) all of the above

1-21. If patients with acute rheumatic fever receive appropriate antibiotic therapy, what percent develop severe cardiac disease (class IV rheumatic heart disease)?

(A) 10 percent
(B) 5 percent
(C) 0.5 percent
(D) 1 percent
(E) none of the above

1-22. The SINGLE MOST important predictor of the outcome of a patient undergoing cardiac surgery is

(A) the pulmonary capillary wedge pressure
(B) the patient's age
(C) the ejection fraction
(D) concomitant disease processes
(E) the end-diastolic left ventricular pressure

1-23. In mitral regurgitation

(A) an amount of blood flows back into the left atrium during diastole
(B) the murmur always radiates into the axilla
(C) patient may have a widely split S2
(D) patient may present with "Corrigan's" pulse
(E) B and C only

1-24. PRIMARILY, diagnosis of valvular heart disease is made by

(A) chest x-ray, arterial blood gases (ABGs), echocardiography, and Doppler
(B) patient history, physical exam, echocardiography, and Doppler
(C) physical exam, cardiac catheterization, ABGs, and echocardiography
(D) physical exam, ejection fraction, loud murmur, Doppler
(E) electrocardiogram (ECG), chest x-ray, echocardiography, cardiac catheterization

1-25. Treatment of valvular heart disease

(A) consists of surgical and nonsurgical
(B) may involve repairing the valve as opposed to replacing the valve
(C) is risky at best
(D) generally has a poor outcome
(E) A and B

1-26. A 69-year-old male presents to the emergency room complaining of sudden onset of severe abdominal pain. A blood pressure of 98/54 is noted and his wife tells you he has been hypertensive for years but never complied with recommended treatment. Abdominal exam reveals a tender, pulsatile, mid-epigastric mass and cool lower extremities with bilateral femoral bruits and diminished pulses. The MOST likely diagnosis is

(A) acute arterial embolus to the lower extremities
(B) perforated gastric ulcer
(C) leaking or ruptured abdominal aneurysm
(D) dissecting thoracic aortic aneurysm

1-27. A 56-year-old obese female smoker with a 10-year history of hypertension awakens one morning with loss of vision in her right eye. This episode resolves spontaneously after 20 min. Later that day, she also notes a "clumsy" right hand. Your exam reveals bilateral carotid bruits, left greater than right. Appropriate management of this patient would include

(A) order noninvasive carotid duplex scans
(B) refer to vascular surgery for possible endarterectomy
(C) unless contraindicated, immediately place the patient on low-dose aspirin
(D) all of the above

1-28. Which of the following statements is TRUE regarding aortic aneurysms?

(A) Patients are commonly asymptomatic.
(B) Aneurysms have a natural history for expanding in size.
(C) Acute arterial insufficiency may be caused by microemboli from an aneurysmal plaque.
(D) all of the above

1-29. A 42-year-old woman describes transient numbness and tingling of her fingers associated with pain and cyanosis upon exposure to cold. You place her hands in cold water and note they turn white, blue, then red after a few minutes. These symptoms are MOST consistent with

(A) thoracic outlet syndrome
(B) transient arteriospasm as seen in Raynaud's disease
(C) atherosclerotic disease of the radial artery
(D) transient vasospasm of the ulnar artery
(E) none of the above

1-30. A 56-year-old diabetic smoker describes progressive "tiredness" and "cramping" in his left calf for 6 to 8 months. Two years ago he jogged 1 to 2 miles every day. Now, walking 5 to 6 blocks or climbing stairs produces leg discomfort that is relieved with 2 to 3 min rest. These symptoms are MOST consistent with

(A) acute arterial insufficiency
(B) deep venous thrombosis
(C) thromboangiitis obliterans (Buerger's disease)
(D) arterial embolus
(E) chronic arterial insufficiency

1-31. All of the following would be appropriate management for chronic arterial insufficiency EXCEPT

(A) low-fat, low-cholesterol diet
(B) smoking cessation and control of hyperglycemia
(C) Trental therapy
(D) exercise regimen with daily walks as tolerated past the point of calf discomfort
(E) warfarin (Coumadin) therapy

1-32. Which of the following is NOT considered a clinical manifestation of acute arterial insufficiency?

(A) pulselessness
(B) paresthesias
(C) paralysis
(D) pyrexia
(E) pain

1-33. Risk factors for developing venous thrombosis include

(A) pregnancy
(B) prolonged bed rest
(C) cancer
(D) IV catheters
(E) all of the above

1-34. Characteristics of deep venous thrombosis include

(A) edema of the extremity proximal to the thrombus
(B) increased risk for embolus to the cerebral vasculature
(C) edema of the extremity distal to the venous occlusion
(D) A and B

1-35. Recommended first-line treatment for femoral vein deep venous thrombosis (DVT) is

(A) urokinase
(B) heparin
(C) warfarin (Coumadin)
(D) aspirin

1. CARDIOVASCULAR

ANSWERS

1-1. The correct answer is D. Peaked T waves occur at around 6 meq/L. As the potassium level rises, the PR interval will elongate and heart block will become evident. Severe hyperkalemia will cause a loss of P waves and a widened QRS. [Singer GG, Brenner BM: Fluid and electrolyte disturbances, in Fauci AS, Braunwald E, Isselbacher KJ, et al (eds): *Harrison's Principles of Internal Medicine,* 14th ed. New York, McGraw-Hill, 1998, pp 265–277.]

1-2. The correct answer is D. In patients presenting with symptoms of cerebral ischemia in more than one territory (i.e., both cerebral hemispheres) the cause is usually due to recurrent emboli, almost always from the heart. Irregular heartbeat and a "subtherapeutic" INR give clues that a patient may be taking warfarin for atrial fibrillation. Atherosclerosis of one of the carotid arteries cannot explain bilateral symptoms. Posterior cerebral ischemia from subclavian steal (or any cause) would rarely produce extremity symptoms; rather it is more commonly associated with dizziness and/or visual changes. Increased intracranial pressure would have a more sudden and dramatic onset. A patient with a normal blood pressure and no change in level of consciousness helps reassure us that hemorrhage is an unlikely etiology. [Diamond MA: Cardiac arrhythmias, in Moser RL (ed): *Primary Care for Physician Assistants.* New York, McGraw-Hill, 1998, chap 1–11.]

1-3. The correct answer is D. A stenosis is said to be "hemodynamically significant" on duplex ultrasonography if it causes changes "downstream" resulting in collateral blood flow. Although such a stenosis may not be causing symptoms per se, it is severe enough to cause changes in the usual flow of blood to the brain and, therefore, should receive further evaluation. A neurologist would be able to gauge the overall risk of stroke in such a patient and begin appropriate medical or surgical therapies. A surgeon with experience in carotid revascularization would also be able to determine if such a patient was appropriate for surgery, or if medical management would be more appropriate. Antiplatelet therapy alone (aspirin, Ticlopidine) would theoretically lower the risk of stroke. CT scan to evaluate for prior infarcts may be done in subsequent workup of a patient with a severe stenosis, but would be of use only to the neurologist or surgeon. The option of yearly follow-up alone, or waiting for symptoms to occur gives a false sense of security and is the least favorable treatment option. Recall that half of all strokes occur without antecedent TIAs. This patient scenario could end with the patient's first symptoms being a devastating or fatal stroke. [Loudenback D: Cerebrovascular accident and transient ischemic attack, in Moser RL (ed): *Primary Care for Physician Assistants.* New York, McGraw-Hill, 1998, chap 1–3.]

1-4. The correct answer is B. Atrial fibrillation is the most common cause of stroke due to cardiac disease. This is due to thrombus that forms in the left atrium, enters the systemic arterial circulation, and travels to the brain resulting in stroke. Atrial fibrillation causes more than half of all cardiogenic emboli, but recent myocardial infarctions cause only about 20 percent. Septal defects and endocarditis are clear risk factors for stroke but only rarely play a role. It is unclear whether mitral valve prolapse poses a significant risk for stroke. [Loudenback D: Cerebrovascular accident and transient ischemic attack, in Moser RL (ed): *Primary Care for Physician Assistants.* New York, McGraw-Hill, 1998, chap 1–3.]

7

1-5. The correct answer is A. Atrial fibrillation is a common cause of *ischemic*, rather than hemorrhagic, stroke. Hypertension is the most important risk factor for primary intracerebral hemorrhage, and cerebral aneurysms are the most common cause of subarachnoid hemorrhage resulting in hemorrhagic stroke. Drugs such as warfarin, as well as illicit drugs, are identified as causes of cerebral hemorrhage. [Loudenback D: Cerebrovascular accident and transient ischemic attack, in Moser RL (ed): *Primary Care for Physician Assistants.* New York, McGraw-Hill, 1998, chap 1–3.]

1-6. The correct answer is E. When dealing with carotid atherosclerosis, the most important piece of information is degree of stenosis. This gives the practitioner the best estimate of risk for a given patient so they can be counseled appropriately. For instance, an asymptomatic stenosis of 30 percent is much less significant for future risk of stroke than a 90 percent stenosis. Vascular surgery is indicated for the symptomatic stenosis or in the asymptomatic stenosis greater than 60 percent in the patient who is an excellent surgical risk, and might benefit over the long term. A CT scan may be useful in the workup for carotid disease, but if the history is unremarkable, it would not be the first step. Neurologists are specialists in the diagnosis and treatment of stroke, but in the asymptomatic patient with a carotid bruit the first step is still determining more about the stenosis itself, and does not require the neurologist's expertise. No treatment at all is always an option, but one cannot know the severity of a carotid plaque simply by physical examination. In patients with evidence for disease in any vascular bed (coronary, peripheral, mesenteric, etc.), a diligent search to rule out disease in other organ systems is crucial. [Mayfield MS: Peripheral vascular disease, in Moser RL (ed): *Primary Care for Physician Assistants.* New York, McGraw-Hill, 1998, chap 1–9.]

1-7. The correct answer is E. Abnormalities of lipid metabolism have several causes. Each of the answers can result in abnormal lipids. [Heymann CJ: Hyperlipidemia, in Moser RL (ed): *Primary Care for Physician Assistants.* New York, McGraw-Hill, 1998, chap 1–6.]

1-8. The correct answer is C. Although all of the medications listed, except aspirin, may be utilized in a lipid-lowering regime, niacin has the broadest spectrum of action and is definitely less expensive than gemfibrozil. ASA is utilized to prevent platelet aggregation. Fiber supplements will aid with constipation and have a minimal effect on lipids. [Heymann CJ: Hyperlipidemia, in Moser RL (ed): *Primary Care for Physician Assistants.* New York, McGraw-Hill, 1998, chap 1–6.]

1-9. The correct answer is E. Each sign or symptom noted is an indication of extreme elevations of either triglycerides or cholesterol. [Heymann CJ: Hyperlipidemia, in Moser RL (ed): *Primary Care for Physician Assistants.* New York, McGraw-Hill, 1998, chap 1–6.]

1-10. The correct answer is C. Cocaine induces intense coronary artery constriction via alpha-adrenergic-sympathetic activity. Using propranolol alone would increase vasoconstriction by the medication's effect in blocking beta sympathetic dilation. Labetalol, a combined alpha and beta blocker, is best to treat the cardiac effects of cocaine. (Willerson JT, Cohn JN: *Cardiovascular Medicine.* New York, Churchill Livingstone, 1995, p 382.)

1-11. The correct answer is C. Typical pulmonary edema in the patient with an acute myocardial infarction is associated with normal central venous pressure (CVP). Pericardial tamponade always increases CVP and classically causes paradoxical pulse. [Sobel BE (ed): *Medical Management of Heart Disease.* New York, Marcel Dekker, 1996, pp 274–276.]

1-12. The correct answer is C. The Framingham Study has demonstrated key risk factors in sudden-death syndrome. In contrast, paroxysmal atrial fibrillation increases risk of stroke. (Kostis JB, Sanders M: *The Prevention of Sudden Cardiac Death*. New York, Wiley-Liss, 1990, pp 1–13.)

1-13.   The correct answer is D.   Unstable angina is due to nonobstructing thrombus in a coronary artery. Therapy is directed toward reducing workload of the heart and reducing platelet stickiness. (Noble J: *Textbook of Primary Care Medicine*. St. Louis, Mosby, 1996, p 231.)

1-14.   The correct answer is E.   Epidemiologic studies have defined risk factors in coronary atherosclerotic heart disease. Changes in diet and cessation of smoking, in addition to modern medicinal therapy, are reducing disease risk. (Braunwald E: *Heart Disease*, 5th ed. Philadelphia, Saunders, 1997, pp 1126–1160.)

1-15.   The correct answer is B.   Myocardial ischemia can be provoked through several diagnostic modalities. These include exercise-induced and pharmacologic-induced techniques. Exercise- or dobutamine-induced ischemia can be diagnosed by demonstration of transient ventricular wall motion abnormalities on the echocardiogram. [Tierney LM Jr, McPhee SJ, Papadakis MA (eds): *Current Medical Diagnosis and Treatment*, 36th ed. Stamford, CT, Appleton & Lange, 1997, pp 324–325.]

1-16.   The correct answer is B.   This young woman, with acute pericarditis, Raynaud's phenomenon, and peripheral neuropathy, has systemic lupus erythematosus. This is an immune-complex disease that also affects the glomerular basement membrane. Remember: Glomerular disease causes microscopic hematuria and proteinuria. [Tierney LM Jr, McPhee SJ, Papadakis MA (eds): *Current Medical Diagnosis and Treatment*, 36th ed. Stamford, CT, Appleton & Lange, 1997, pp 774–777.]

1-17.   The correct answer is C.   Recent epidemiologic studies have documented the strong beneficial effect of warfarin in reducing the incidence of stroke in high-risk atrial fibrillation patients. Warfarin is to be prescribed in patients with and without underlying structural heart disease unless contraindication exists. (Cohen IS, Ezekowitz MD: Prevention of thromboembolism in patients with atrial fibrillation. *Cardiol Clin* 14:537, 1996.)

1-18.   The correct answer is A.   Total cholesterol is important, but LDL-C is felt to be the most atherogenic. HDL-C is protective against atherosclerosis and elevations are beneficial. The exact role of triglycerides and chylomicrons in atherogenesis is not clearly defined. [Heymann CJ: Atherosclerosis, in Moser RL (ed): *Primary Care for Physician Assistants*. New York, McGraw-Hill, 1998, chap 1–4.]

1-19.   The correct answer is C.   Heavily calcified plaque is more stable and ruptures less frequently than soft, cholesterol-filled plaque. Vessel occlusion of up to 90 percent can maintain adequate blood flow to distal tissues. Vasospasm may cause signs and symptoms of ischemia but is a temporary, not a physiologic, change. [Diamond MA: Ischemic coronary artery syndromes, in Moser RL (ed): *Primary Care for Physician Assistants*. New York, McGraw-Hill, 1998, chap 1–7.]

1-20.   The correct answer is E.   Benefits of serum lipid reduction are multidimensional and have significant metabolic impact on atherosclerotic vascular disease. [Heymann CJ: Hyperlipidemia, in Moser RL (ed): *Primary Care for Physician Assistants*. New York, McGraw-Hill, 1998, chap 1–6.]

1-21.   The correct answer is D.   If patients with acute rheumatic fever receive appropriate prophylactic antibiotic therapy, about 1 percent develop severe (class IV) cardiac disease and 4 percent develop debilitating rheumatic heart disease. [Smith JR: Acquired valvular heart disease, in Moser RL (ed): *Primary Care for Physician Assistants*. New York, McGraw-Hill, 1998, chap 1–10.]

1-22. The correct answer is C. The single most important predictor of outcome in a patient undergoing cardiac surgery is the ejection fraction. [Diamond MA: Ischemic coronary artery syndromes, in Moser RL (ed): *Primary Care for Physician Assistants.* New York, McGraw-Hill, 1998, chap 1–7.]

1-23. The correct answer is C. One of the findings on physical exam may include a widely split S2. In mitral regurgitation, blood flows back into the left atrium during systole. Corrigan's pulse is commonly noted in aortic regurgitation. In the case of a posterior leaflet chordae tendineae rupture, a murmur that mimics aortic stenosis may be found. [Smith JR: Acquired valvular heart disease, in Moser RL (ed): *Primary Care for Physician Assistants.* New York, McGraw-Hill, 1998, chap 1–10.]

1-24. The correct answer is A. The history and physical exam remain the cornerstone for diagnosis of acquired valvular heart disease. Radiographic studies such as echocardiography and color-flow Doppler studies confirm the diagnosis and provide vital information with regard to severity of disease. [Smith JR: Acquired valvular heart disease, in Moser RL (ed): *Primary Care for Physician Assistants.* New York, McGraw-Hill, 1998, chap 1–10.]

1-25. The correct answer is E. The two basic approaches to treatment of valvular heart disease are either surgical or nonsurgical. Of the surgical options, repair of the valve may be advantageous over replacement. [Smith JR: Acquired valvular heart disease, in Moser RL (ed): *Primary Care for Physician Assistants.* New York, McGraw-Hill, 1998, chap 1–10.]

1-26. The correct answer is C. Sudden abdominal pain, a pulsatile abdominal mass, hypotension, and signs of decreased perfusion to the lower extremity are classic findings associated with a leaking or ruptured abdominal aneurysm. Manifestations of shock may also occur with gastric perforation or thoracic aortic dissection. However, additional findings (i.e., pulsatile abdominal mass, vascular bruits, and diminished pulses) are atypical for these disorders. Arterial embolus would present with symptoms of severe limb pain, pallor, and sudden loss of pulses. [Mayfield MS: Peripheral vascular disease, in Moser RL (ed): *Primary Care for Physician Assistants.* New York, McGraw-Hill, 1998, chap 1–9.]

1-27. The correct answer is D. Symptoms described are classic for transient ischemic attack, a precursor for ischemic strokes. The presence of amaurosis fugax (transient monocular blindness) supports the involvement of the ophthalmic branch off the carotid artery. A carotid duplex scan is warranted to look for concomitant occlusive disease of the carotid artery. Aspirin has antiplatelet activity and is a therapeutic adjuvant to prevent recurrent ischemic events. A carotid endarterectomy should be considered in selected patients with TIAs due to impaired carotid circulation to prevent future stroke. [Loudenback D: Cerebrovascular accident and transient ischemic attack, in Moser RL (ed): *Primary Care for Physician Assistants.* New York, McGraw-Hill, 1998, chap 1–3.]

1-28. The correct answer is D. Small, stable aneurysms typically do not cause symptoms. Aneurysms, however, tend to increase in size over time and most will eventually rupture. A thrombotic plaque may form along the luminal wall of an aneurysm, fragment, and embolize, producing symptoms of acute arterial insufficiency. [Mayfield MS: Peripheral vascular disease, in Moser RL (ed): *Primary Care for Physician Assistants.* New York, McGraw-Hill, 1998, chap 1–9.]

1-29. The correct answer is B. A triphasic color change of the digits after exposure to cold is classic for Raynaud's disease. Color changes are caused by the effects of transient arteriospasm. Thoracic outlet syndrome is a neurovascular condition caused by compression of the brachial plexus, subclavian artery, or subclavian vein at the thoracic outlet located inferior to the clavicle. Patients typically complain of pain, paresthesias, and weakness of the upper extremity or neck and shoulder. Symptoms of arterial insufficiency are less common. Symptoms caused by atherosclerotic occlusive disease of the upper extremity or ulnar artery vasospasm are rare. [Mayfield MS: Peripheral vascular disease, in Moser RL (ed): *Primary Care for Physician Assistants*. New York, McGraw-Hill, 1998, chap 1–9.]

1-30. **The correct answer is E.** Exercise-induced calf discomfort that is relieved with brief periods of rest is classic for claudication, a primary symptom of chronic arterial insufficiency. Acute arterial occlusion is manifested as acute onset of continuous, severe limb pain distal to the site of vascular occlusion. Thromboangiitis obliterans typically presents as digital ischemia. Arterial embolism to the distal extremity commonly manifests as symptoms of acute arterial insufficiency. [Mayfield MS: Peripheral vascular disease, in Moser RL (ed): *Primary Care for Physician Assistants*. New York, McGraw-Hill, 1998, chap 1–9.]

1-31. **The correct answer is E.** Treatment for chronic arterial insufficiency includes reduction of modifiable risk factors for atherosclerosis (smoking, high-fat/high-cholesterol diet, hypertension, and diabetes). A daily exercise program that includes walking past the point of claudication would enhance the development of collateral circulation. Trental is a medication that enhances the ability of red cells to pass through stenotic vessels and may improve claudication in some patients. Warfarin (Coumadin) is used for long-term management and prevention of recurrent acute arterial insufficiency that is embolic in origin. [Mayfield MS: Peripheral vascular disease, in Moser RL (ed): *Primary Care for Physician Assistants*. New York, McGraw-Hill, 1998, chap 1–9.]

1-32. **The correct answer is D.** The five P's for acute arterial insufficiency are pain, pulselessness, pallor, paresthesias, and paralysis. Pyrexia (fever) is not a common associated finding. [Mayfield MS: Peripheral vascular disease, in Moser RL (ed): *Primary Care for Physician Assistants*. New York, McGraw-Hill, 1998, chap 1–9.]

1-33. **The correct answer is E.** Any process that produces venous stasis (prolonged immobilization or pregnancy), injury to the vessel wall (IV catheters), or a hypercoagulable state (cancer) can precipitate the formation of intraluminal venous clots. [Mayfield MS: Peripheral vascular disease, in Moser RL (ed): *Primary Care for Physician Assistants*. New York, McGraw-Hill, 1998, chap 1–9.]

1-34. **The correct answer is C.** Emboli from the venous circulation will be carried to the right side of the heart and subsequently the pulmonary vascular bed. Cerebral vessels are not affected by venous emboli. A venous thrombus will obstruct blood return to the vena cava and heart resulting in edema that is distal to the site of vessel occlusion. [Mayfield MS: Peripheral vascular disease, in Moser RL (ed): *Primary Care for Physician Assistants*. New York, McGraw-Hill, 1998, chap 1–9.]

1-35. **The correct answer is B.** Urokinase is more commonly used to lyse arterial clots. Warfarin (Coumadin) may be used to initiate treatment of calf vein DVTs and for continued outpatient therapy for DVTs of larger or more proximal vessels. Aspirin may be effective adjuvant therapy for thrombotic or embolic arterial occlusive disease. Recommended treatment for popliteal or iliofemoral DVT is intravenous heparin titrated to maintain the APTT at 1.5 to 2 times normal. [Mayfield MS: Peripheral vascular disease, in Moser RL (ed): *Primary Care for Physician Assistants*. New York, McGraw-Hill, 1998, chap 1–9.]

SECTION 2
DERMATOLOGY

2. DERMATOLOGY

QUESTIONS

DIRECTIONS: Each question below contains suggested responses. Choose the **one best** response to each question.

2-1. All the following statements about seborrheic keratoses are TRUE EXCEPT

(A) They vary quite a bit in appearance.
(B) They are uncommon.
(C) Around eyes, they tend to be soft and pedunculated.
(D) Palms and soles are unaffected by seborrheic keratoses.

2-2. The development of seborrheic keratoses is related to

(A) an inherited familial tendency
(B) sun exposure
(C) friction and trauma
(D) a viral infection

2-3. The sudden (in days to weeks) appearance of multiple seborrheic keratoses in a previously unaffected individual who has an occult internal malignancy is called

(A) the Koebner phenomenon
(B) the isomorphic phenomenon
(C) papulosa nigra
(D) the Leser-Trelat sign

2-4. Valid arguments in favor of yeast causation of seborrheic dermatitis include which ONE of the following?

(A) Seborrheic dermatitis patients tend to be diabetic.
(B) Seborrheic dermatitis occurs only where *Pityrosporum* thrives.
(C) Histologic sections through affected follicles show increased numbers of yeast organisms.
(D) Seborrheic dermatitis worsens dramatically with HIV disease.

2-5. A 60-year-old man presents with seborrheic dermatitis of relatively rapid onset affecting mostly the face. During this time, he has begun to walk with a shuffling gait. It is quite possible, judging from this history, that this man has

(A) Parkinson's disease
(B) HIV disease
(C) multiple myeloma
(D) alcoholic dementia

2-6. Which ONE of the following statements about seborrheic dermatitis is TRUE?

(A) Seborrheic dermatitis is a chronic, incurable condition.
(B) Seborrheic dermatitis is not associated with any serious disease.
(C) Seborrheic dermatitis only affects the face.
(D) Seborrheic dermatitis is caused by yeast organisms.

2-7. Adult seborrheic dermatitis affects all of the following areas EXCEPT

(A) midinterscapular area
(B) eyes/eyelids
(C) anterior tibial skin
(D) umbilical skin

2-8. A 68-year-old white male presents to the office with a lesion on his left lower lip that has been present for 8 months. It has gotten larger since he first noticed it. The lesion is ulcerated with partial crusting and nontender. He has a 50-pack/year smoking history. The MOST likely diagnosis is

(A) squamous cell carcinoma
(B) cheilitis
(C) basal cell carcinoma
(D) solar keratosis

2-9. Which of the following viruses has been associated with the development of squamous cell carcinoma?

(A) poxvirus
(B) human papillomavirus
(C) herpes simplex virus
(D) enterovirus

2-10. Which of the following skin lesion(s) is/are pre-cancerous?

(A) leukoplakia
(B) actinic keratosis
(C) neither A nor B
(D) both A and B

2-11. The possible treatment of squamous cell carcinoma may include all the following EXCEPT

(A) surgery plus radiation
(B) surgical excision alone
(C) radiation alone
(D) chemotherapy

2-12. Which of the following lesions has a high incidence of later conversion to malignant melanoma?

(A) blue nevus
(B) seborrheic keratosis
(C) congenital nevomelanocytic nevus (hairy nevus)
(D) brown nevus
(E) acrochordon

2-13. All of the following are types of malignant melanoma EXCEPT

(A) acrolentiginous
(B) desmoplastic
(C) nodular
(D) superficial spreading
(E) lentigo-maligna

2-14. All of the following are descriptions of a malignant melanoma lesion EXCEPT

(A) multiple colors
(B) asymmetric
(C) itching
(D) irregular borders
(E) diameter >5 mm

2-15. All of the following are considered when staging malignant melanoma EXCEPT

(A) involvement thickness
(B) extension
(C) lymph node involvement
(D) organ
(E) location

2-16. All of the following are considered risk factors for development of malignant melanoma EXCEPT

(A) a family history of malignant melanoma
(B) a history of blistering sunburn
(C) fair skin and red hair
(D) personal history of squamous cell carcinoma of the skin
(E) poor tanning capacity

2-17. Which of the following is the MOST common type of skin cancer?

(A) malignant melanoma
(B) squamous cell carcinoma
(C) basal cell carcinoma
(D) actinic keratosis

2-18. All of the following describe a basal cell carcinoma of the skin EXCEPT

(A) nonhealing papule
(B) nonhealing ulcer
(C) painful lesion
(D) infrequently bleeding lesion

2-19. All of the following are possible treatments of basal cell carcinoma of the skin EXCEPT

(A) surgical excision
(B) cryotherapy
(C) laser eradication
(D) electrodesiccation
(E) chemotherapy

2-20. Which of the following terms may be used to describe a basal cell carcinoma?

(A) rodent ulcer
(B) telangiectatic keratosis
(C) umbilicus ulcer
(D) "pancake" ulcer

2-21. Risk factors for the development of basal cell carcinoma of the skin include all the following EXCEPT

(A) fair skin with poor tanning capacity
(B) previous x-ray therapy for acne
(C) outside occupations
(D) dark skin
(E) frequent use of tanning booths

2-22. Condyloma acuminata can be treated with which of the following?

(A) podophyllin
(B) Efudex
(C) trichloroacetic acid
(D) interferon alpha
(E) all of the above

2-23. Treatment for verruca plana includes which of the following?

(A) Retin A
(B) Efudex
(C) cryotherapy
(D) A and C
(E) all of the above

2-24. Which of the following is known to cause hand-foot-and-mouth disease?

(A) poxvirus
(B) *Treponema pallidum*
(C) coxsackievirus
(D) human papillomavirus

2-25. Hand-foot-and-mouth disease has discrete vesicular lesions on the palms and soles. Which of the following is also known to have a rash on the palms and soles?

(A) herpes simplex
(B) Rocky Mountain spotted fever
(C) meningococcemia
(D) scarlatina

2-26. Which of the following is an accurate description of the oral lesions seen in hand-foot-and-mouth disease?

(A) pus-filled vesicles on the tongue that are >5 mm in diameter
(B) small white-to-gray vesicles in the pharynx with a red halo
(C) numerous vesicles on the oral mucosa that coalesce into large flaccid bullae
(D) ulcers on the buccal mucosa, but no vesicles

2-27. Which ONE of the following causes molluscum contagiosum?

(A) poxvirus
(B) herpesvirus
(C) human papillomavirus
(D) enterovirus
(E) rotavirus

2-28. A significant number of large facial molluscum contagiosum nodules may be associated with which of the following?

(A) HPV infection
(B) HIV infection
(C) infancy
(D) shaving

2-29. Which of the following is a differential diagnosis of molluscum contagiosum?

(A) condylomata lata
(B) verruca vulgaris
(C) condylomata acuminata
(D) basal cell carcinoma

2-30. In distinguishing between a plantar wart and a simple callus, all of the following statements are TRUE EXCEPT

(A) A wart is most tender to direct pressure.
(B) Skin lines do not go through the lesion.
(C) There is pinpoint bleeding when the lesion is debrided.
(D) A KOH is useless in helping determine the presence of a wart.
(E) Plantar warts may be in weight-bearing or non–weight-bearing areas.

2-31. Plantar warts are difficult to treat because

(A) they are very deep and have roots into the dermis
(B) they are caused by a bacteria that is resistant to treatment
(C) they usually are singular lesions
(D) the epidermis is very thick on the bottom of the foot and hard to penetrate with medication
(E) they look like foreign-body reactions

2-32. Ingrown toenails

(A) are best treated by cutting a V in the center of the nail
(B) are frequently caused by improper nail trimming
(C) should initially be dug out by the patient
(D) occur only on the medial and lateral borders of the nail
(E) should usually be treated with oral antibiotics

2-33. The etiologic agent of bullous impetigo is

(A) group A beta-hemolytic *Streptococci*
(B) *Staphylococcus aureus*
(C) *Pseudomonas aeruginosa*
(D) A and B
(E) none of the above

2-34. Which of the following treatment options are appropriate for impetigo?

(A) mupirocin ointment (Bactroban)
(B) penicillin
(C) erythromycin
(D) ciprofloxacin
(E) none of the above

2-35. Which of the following statements is FALSE regarding impetigo?

(A) *Staphylococcus aureus* is present in the nasal passages, axillae, and perineum of 20 percent of adults.

(B) The antistreptolysin titer (ASO) rises significantly after group A beta-hemolytic streptococcal infection and is a sensitive indicator of streptococcal impetigo.

(C) Flares of guttate psoriasis can be precipitated by streptococcal impetigo.

(D) The majority of patients who develop acute glomerulonephritis improve within 1 to 2 weeks.

(E) The most common clinical features of acute glomerulonephritis include hematuria, proteinuria, edema, and hypertension.

2-36. All the following statements about lichen planus are TRUE EXCEPT

(A) Lichen planus is usually difficult to diagnose.

(B) A basic lichen planus lesion is papular.

(C) Lichen planus lesions are often distinctively purple.

(D) Lichen planus can affect oral mucosa.

2-37. The classically described "P's" of lichen planus include all of the following EXCEPT

(A) planar (meaning flat-topped)

(B) penile (and of course, vulvar)

(C) pruritic (though 20 percent don't itch)

(D) perioral (i.e., around the mouth)

2-38. Which of the following are accepted treatment options for pityriasis rosea?

(A) a group V topical steroid

(B) oral antihistamines

(C) UVB phototherapy

(D) no treatment is required, as this is a self-limited disease

(E) all of the above

2-39. Which of the following laboratory tests can assist in making the diagnosis of pityriasis rosea?

(A) a KOH of a skin scraping can rule out fungal infections

(B) a skin biopsy is always warranted in cases of suspected pityriasis rosea

(C) an RPR should be considered in sexually active individuals

(D) A and C

(E) all of the above

2-40. Tinea versicolor is caused by which of the following organisms?

(A) *Pityrosporum*

(B) *Microsporum*

(C) *Trichophyton*

(D) *Epidermophyton*

2-41. A 19-year-old white male presents to your office for an initial visit with complaints of itching and burning of the feet and maceration of the skin between the toes. Which of the following historical statements would be MOST helpful to you in developing your differential diagnosis?

(A) history of exposure to *Rhus* plant species

(B) a family member with the same symptoms

(C) daily use of dark-colored socks

(D) participation in school athletics with daily practice sessions

2-42. Which of the following office procedures assists in the immediate diagnosis of a tinea infection?

(A) fungal culture

(B) saline wet mount

(C) bacterial culture

(D) 10% KOH preparation

2-43. Regarding treatment of scalp psoriasis, choose the ONE correct statement from among the following

(A) Scalp psoriasis is no more difficult to treat than psoriasis in other areas of the body.

(B) Scalp psoriasis is relatively asymptomatic compared to psoriasis on the rest of the body.

(C) Scalp psoriasis seldom results in hair loss.

(D) Scalp psoriasis almost never occurs without signs of psoriasis elsewhere.

2-44. A psoriatic patient presents with complaint of his usual topical steroid preparation becoming less and less effective. MOST likely, this is a phenomenon called

(A) Woronoff's

(B) tachyphylaxis

(C) Auspitz's

(D) Munro's

2-45. The treatment of choice for scabies in infants under 6 months of age and pregnant women is

(A) permethrin 5% cream

(B) lindane 1% lotion

(C) crotamiton 10% cream

(D) sulfur 6 to 10% ointment

(E) none of the above

2-46. Which ONE of the following statements is TRUE regarding arthropod infestations?

(A) Pubic lice are almost always due to poor patient hygiene.

(B) Secondary bacterial infections occurring after anthropod infestations can be adequately treated with topical mupirocin.

(C) Ivermectin 200 μg/kg orally one-time dose is the treatment of choice for scabies in the immunocompetent host.

(D) Rheumatic fever has been reported after secondary infection of lesions with group A beta-hemolytic streptococci.

(E) Acute glomerulonephritis has been reported after secondary infection of lesions with *Staphylococcus aureus*.

2-47. With regard to the treatment of atopic dermatitis, all the following statements are TRUE EXCEPT

(A) Antibiotics are frequently used in refractory cases.

(B) Frequent moisturization is a key factor in treating atopic dermatitis.

(C) Prednisone or other systemic corticosteroids are frequently used for atopic dermatitis.

(D) Patient and/or family education about atopic dermatitis is essential.

2-48. Bullous pemphigoid is characterized by

(A) a benign course
(B) a positive Nikolsky's sign
(C) easily ruptured blisters
(D) symmetrical involvement of limbs

2-49. Relatively common dermatoses that can present with bullae include all the following EXCEPT

(A) molluscum contagiosum
(B) lichen planus
(C) insect bites
(D) pityriasis rosea

2-50. An indolent cellulitic process involving the hands of those occupationally engaged in handling fish, poultry, and meat would MOST likely be

(A) necrotizing fasciitis
(B) cryptococcal cellulitis
(C) erysipelas
(D) erysipeloid cellulitis

2-51. Which of the following causes the reaction of rhus dermatitis?

(A) the oleoresin on the plant
(B) the vesicular fluid of an affected individual
(C) exposure to English ivy
(D) insect bites

2-52. Which of the following materials used to make jewelry will commonly cause contact dermatitis in sensitive individuals?

(A) sapphire
(B) silver
(C) gold
(D) nickel/chromium
(E) titanium

2-53. The dressing for a pressure ulcer should

(A) adhere firmly and dry quickly
(B) keep the ulcer moist and the surrounding tissue dry
(C) keep the ulcer tissue dry and the surrounding tissue moist
(D) keep both the ulcer and surrounding tissue moist

2-54. A patient presents with obvious erythema multiforme minor. Looking for a likely trigger, your initial history taking should include questioning about (choose the ONE best answer)

(A) the patient's stress level
(B) excessive sun exposure
(C) exposure to cats
(D) recent HSV I or II attack

2-55. A 26-year-old woman presents with an obvious case of erythema nodosum. Initial history taking should include questions about (choose the ONE BEST answer)

(A) her stress level
(B) any new medications she may have started
(C) history of foreign travel
(D) insect bites to the legs

2-56. The bilateral hilar adenopathy often found on the chest x-rays of erythema nodosum patients (choose the ONE statement that BEST completes the sentence)

(A) means the patient likely has lymphoma
(B) indicates that sarcoidosis is the trigger
(C) is a common, benign finding in erythema nodosum patients
(D) means the patient likely has tuberculosis

2-57.   The treatment of erythema nodosum should include

(A) broad-spectrum antibiotics
(B) topical steroids
(C) finding and eliminating the trigger if possible
(D) systemic steroids

2-58.   A 15-year-old boy presents with an as yet un-explained, painless but dramatic swelling of the upper lip. The likely diagnosis is

(A) cellulitis
(B) hereditary angioedema (HAE)
(C) contact dermatitis
(D) angioedema

2-59.   Initial treatment of common furuncles of acute onset should include all of the following EXCEPT

(A) systemic antibiotics
(B) hot compresses
(C) incision and drainage, as indicated
(D) elimination of known etiologic factors

2-60.   A family of three presents with lesions and a history strongly suggestive of *Pseudomonas folliculitis* ("hot-tub folliculitis"). Assuming a correct diagnosis, you would (choose ONE correct answer)

(A) reassure them about the self-limited nature of the problem and refer them to county health department for advice on how to prevent future problems
(B) prescribe mupirocin ointment for topical use and oral Cipro 500 mg bid × 10 days
(C) try to identify and treat all contacts since this is highly contagious
(D) incise and drain each pustule

2. DERMATOLOGY

ANSWERS

2-1. The correct answer is B. Seborrheic keratoses are, in fact, the most common benign skin lesions. The others are true statements, and point to the fact that seborrheic keratoses are found on most areas of the body and can vary greatly in appearance, depending on location. [Monroe J: Seborrheic keratosis, in Moser RL (ed): *Primary Care for Physician Assistants.* New York, McGraw-Hill, 1998, chap 2–26.]

2-2. The correct answer is A. Early onset of these lesions (before age 25) is not uncommon, and itself seems to be an inherited trait. Seborrheic keratoses development does not appear to be related to sun exposure (B), nor is it related to trauma or friction (C). Finally, even though seborrheic keratoses can be very similar in appearance to warts, their development is not related to any viral infection (D). Advancing age seems to be the other major factor in acquiring these lesions. [Monroe J: Seborrheic keratosis, in Moser RL (ed): *Primary Care for Physician Assistants.* New York, McGraw-Hill, 1998, chap 2–26.]

2-3. The correct answer is D. The Leser-Trelat sign is thought by some to be a variant of another paraneoplastic sign called acanthosis nigricans. This is the only known serious implication of having seborrheic keratoses. The Koebner phenomenon (A) is the name for trauma-provoked lesion configurations, as with psoriasis or warts. This term is synonymous with the isomorphic phenomenon (B). Papulosa nigra (C) is the name given to seborrheic keratosis–like papules that most often develop on the faces of African-Americans. [Monroe J: Seborrheic keratosis, in Moser RL (ed): *Primary Care for Physician Assistants.* New York, McGraw-Hill, 1998, chap 2–26.]

2-4. The correct answer is D, and is seen by some as prime evidence of their theory of seborrheic dermatitis being caused by this organism. Seborrheic dermatitis has no known connection with diabetes, so A is an incorrect choice. Seborrheic dermatitis also occurs in areas where there are few *P. ovale* organisms found, such as in the axillae, so B is an incorrect choice. Histologic sections have failed to show increased numbers of yeast organisms, so C is an incorrect statement. [Monroe J: Seborrheic dermatitis, in Moser RL (ed): *Primary Care for Physician Assistants.* New York, McGraw-Hill, 1998, chap 2–25.]

2-5. The correct answer is A. For unknown reasons, the seborrheic areas of the face (nasolabial folds primarily) become more oily with Parkinson's, and this is thought to be responsible for the seborrheic dermatitis one sees as this disease progresses. Seborrheic dermatitis can dramatically worsen with HIV, but the latter is not associated with gait disturbances until the latter stages of the disease, if at all, so B is an incorrect choice. Multiple myeloma (C) is not associated with seborrheic dermatitis. Seborrheic dermatitis is a bit more common in alcoholics, but this combination is not likely to explain the clinical picture as given, so D is an incorrect choice. [Monroe J: Seborrheic dermatitis, in Moser RL (ed): *Primary Care for Physician Assistants.* New York, McGraw-Hill, 1998, chap 2–25.]

2-6. The correct answer is A. It's important for patients to understand this; otherwise, any treatment will "fail," i.e., not cure them. B is an incorrect statement because seborrheic dermatitis can herald the arrival of diseases such as HIV, Parkinson's, or Leiner's. C is incorrect because seborrheic dermatitis can be found in a number of nonfacial areas, including groin, sternal skin, and back. It is true that it most commonly affects the face. D is not a statement that can be proven, even though some prominent dermatologists believe it to be true. Most of the experts are still undecided about the etiology of seborrheic dermatitis. [Monroe J: Seborrheic dermatitis, in Moser RL (ed): *Primary Care for Physician Assistants*. New York, McGraw-Hill, 1998, chap 2–25.]

2-7. The correct answer is C. Anterior tibial skin has a relative lack of sebaceous glands. Seborrheic dermatitis does occasionally affect the interscapular skin (A), does cause blepharoconjunctivitis and styes in some unlucky individuals (B), and is well known to present with a florid, red, occasionally weepy rash involving the umbilicus (D). [Monroe J: Seborrheic dermatitis, in Moser RL (ed): *Primary Care for Physician Assistants*. New York, McGraw-Hill, 1998, chap 2–25.]

2-8. The correct answer is A. Squamous cell carcinoma forms on the lower lip of heavy or long-term smokers, where they rest their cigarette. It is likely due to chronic exposure to the chemicals in cigarettes. Cheilitis is inflammation and cracking at the corners of the mouth and may be from a nutritional deficiency or chronic chapping. Basal cell carcinoma presents as a hard, nodular lesion with rolled, elevated edges. This does not usually ulcerate. Solar keratosis appears as a dark, waxy, elevated lesion that appears "stuck on" the skin. This lesion is benign and is not due to cigarette smoking. [Sauls BL: Squamous cell carcinoma, in Moser RL (ed): *Primary Care for Physician Assistants*. New York, McGraw-Hill, 1998, chap 2–27.]

2-9. The correct answer is B. Human papillomavirus causes development of condylomata acuminata infection of the cervix, penis, and anal area. Certain subtypes of this virus predispose an individual to later development of squamous cell carcinoma in the same area. Eradication of the wart-like lesions does not eliminate the virus from the system. Herpes simplex virus causes painful vesicular lesions but does not predispose the individual to the future development of skin cancer. Both poxvirus and enterovirus are generic group names for many viruses that cause various skin, GI, and other infections, none of which predispose to squamous cell carcinoma. [Sauls BL: Squamous cell carcinoma, in Moser RL (ed): *Primary Care for Physician Assistants*. New York, McGraw-Hill, 1998, chap 2–27.]

2-10. The correct answer is D. Actinic keratoses are hyperpigmented scaly skin lesions commonly found on sun-exposed areas, especially the tops of the hands and the face. These lesions routinely turn into squamous cell carcinoma unless treated. Appropriate treatment includes surgical excision and topical 5-FU (fluorouracil) cream. Leukoplakia is a smooth white patch found on mucous membranes of the buccal mucosa and female perineal area. This lesion is often precancerous and a biopsy should be taken when first noted. [Sauls BL: Squamous cell carcinoma, in Moser RL (ed): *Primary Care for Physician Assistants*. New York, McGraw-Hill, 1998, chap 2–27.]

2-11. The correct answer is D. The treatment of squamous cell carcinoma usually consists of either surgical excision or radiation alone depending on many factors, including the size and location of the lesion and the age of the patient as well as their current condition. Some cases may require a combination of both therapies. Chemotherapy is not used in the treatment of squamous cell carcinoma. [Sauls BL: Squamous cell carcinoma, in Moser RL (ed): *Primary Care for Physician Assistants*. New York, McGraw-Hill, 1998, chap 2–27.]

2-12. The correct answer is C. Congenital nevomelanocytic (hairy) nevi have a great propensity for conversion to malignant melanoma later in life. Individuals born with these lesions should have early evaluation and lesion removal. Brown and blue nevi are benign lesions that are not known to have frequent malignant conversion. Seborrheic keratoses are dark, waxy, stuck-on lesions that occur in mid- to late life. They are not premalignant and do not require treatment. Acrochordons are skin tags. These are also benign and do not require treatment. [Sauls BL: Malignant melanoma, in Moser RL (ed): *Primary Care for Physician Assistants*. New York, McGraw-Hill, 1998, chap 2–21.]

2-13. The correct answer is B. Desmoplastic refers to a type of nevi. The four types of malignant melanoma are acrolentiginous, nodular, lentigo-maligna, and superficial spreading. The last one is the most commonly seen, especially in Caucasians. [Sauls BL: Malignant melanoma, in Moser RL (ed): *Primary Care for Physician Assistants*. New York, McGraw-Hill, 1998, chap 2–21.]

2-14. The correct answer is C. The typical malignant melanoma lesion has one or more of the ABCDES elements: asymmetry, border irregularity, multiple colors, diameter >5 mm, elevation, and shadowing. Any of these may signify development of malignant melanoma and warrants biopsy. [Sauls BL: Malignant melanoma, in Moser RL (ed): *Primary Care for Physician Assistants*. New York, McGraw-Hill, 1998, chap 2–21.]

2-15. The correct answer is E. Typical staging for malignant melanoma includes thickness of the lesion, extension into surrounding tissue, local and distant lymph node involvement, and organ involvement. Widespread disease is generally incurable and treatment consists of palliative measures such as radiation. Excision is reserved for small localized lesions. Other patients may be candidates for chemotherapy or immunotherapy. [Sauls BL: Malignant melanoma, in Moser RL (ed): *Primary Care for Physician Assistants*. New York, McGraw-Hill, 1998, chap 2–21.]

2-16. The correct answer is D. A personal history of squamous cell carcinoma or basal cell carcinoma of the skin does not predispose one to malignant melanoma, though previous malignant melanoma is obviously significant. Fair-skinned individuals with poor tanning capacity are at highest risk. A history of one to three blistering sunburns, even as a child, has been statistically correlated with later formation of melanoma. [Sauls BL: Malignant melanoma, in Moser RL (ed): *Primary Care for Physician Assistants*. New York, McGraw-Hill, 1998, chap 2–21.]

2-17. The correct answer is C. The most common type of skin cancer is basal cell carcinoma, which arises in epidermal basal cells. These are slow-growing lesions that rarely metastasize. Squamous cell carcinoma is the second most common cancer. Malignant melanoma is the rarest. Actinic keratosis is a premalignant lesion of the skin, not a skin cancer. [Sauls BL: Basal cell carcinoma, in Moser RL (ed): *Primary Care for Physician Assistants*. New York, McGraw-Hill, 1998, chap 2–7.]

2-18. The correct answer is C. Basal cell carcinomas of the skin are described as slowly evolving, nonhealing papular, nodular, or ulcerated lesions that are not painful and rarely bleed. The borders of these lesions are often described as having a "rolled edge." Metastases are uncommon with these lesions. [Sauls BL: Basal cell carcinoma, in Moser RL (ed): *Primary Care for Physician Assistants*. New York, McGraw-Hill, 1998, chap 2–7.]

2-19. The correct answer is E. Basal cell carcinoma of the skin is most commonly treated with surgical excision. Alternative therapies include laser eradication, cryotherapy, and electrocautery. Chemotherapy is not used in the treatment of basal cell carcinoma. The cure rate is high if treated early. [Sauls BL: Basal cell carcinoma, in Moser RL (ed): *Primary Care for Physician Assistants*. New York, McGraw-Hill, 1998, chap 2–7.]

2-20. The correct answer is A. Basal cell carcinomas of the skin often evolve into nonhealing ulcerated areas, hence the name "rodent ulcer." [Sauls BL: Basal cell carcinoma, in Moser RL (ed): *Primary Care for Physician Assistants*. New York, McGraw-Hill, 1998, chap 2–7.]

2-21. **The correct answer is D.** Basal cell carcinoma occurs most commonly on areas of the body that have been frequently exposed to the sun. UV radiation damages the skin, so previous x-ray therapy also causes some amount of skin damage and may predispose to future development of this cancer. Occupations that are outside, such as farming, road work, house building, etc., also predispose the person to skin cancer. Dark skin is protective against UV radiation, and individuals having such skin have a lower incidence of skin cancers. [Sauls BL: Basal cell carcinoma, in Moser RL (ed): *Primary Care for Physician Assistants*. New York, McGraw-Hill, 1998, chap 2–7.]

2-22. **The correct answer is E.** Condyloma acuminata can be treated with any one or combination of the following: topical podophyllin preparations, topical trichloroacetic acid, cryotherapy, electrocautery, surgical or laser excision, oral cimetidine, intralesional interferon alpha, topical 5-fluorouracil. [DiBaise M: Human papillomavirus, in Moser RL (ed): *Primary Care for Physician Assistants*. New York, McGraw-Hill, 1998, chap 2–18.]

2-23. **The correct answer is E.** Verruca plana can be treated with any one or combination of the following: topical tretinoin (Retin A), topical 5-fluorouracil, and cryotherapy. [DiBaise M: Human papillomavirus, in Moser RL (ed): *Primary Care for Physician Assistants*. New York, McGraw-Hill, 1998, chap 2–18.]

2-24. **The correct answer is C.** Hand-foot-and-mouth disease is associated with infection by subtype A16 of the coxsackievirus family. Poxvirus causes molluscum contagiosum. *Treponema pallidum* is a spirochete that causes syphilis. Human papillomavirus causes condylomata acuminata (genital warts). [Sauls BL: Hand-foot-and-mouth disease, in Moser RL (ed): *Primary Care for Physician Assistants*. New York, McGraw-Hill, 1998, chap 2–15.]

2-25. **The correct answer is B.** Rocky Mountain spotted fever is one of the differential diagnoses of hand-foot-and-mouth disease due to the occurrence of the palm and sole rash that is uncommon in most viral and bacterial infections. Rocky Mountain spotted fever differs in that there is also a prominent rash on the trunk and extremities, which is absent in hand-foot-and-mouth disease. Meningococcemia is a life-threatening illness that often manifests with dark purplish purpura on the extremities along with meningeal signs. Scarlatina (also known as scarlet fever) is a sandpaper-like rash seen with a streptococcal infection. Herpes simplex causes painful vesicles and ulcers that occur on the oral or genital mucosa. [Sauls BL: Hand-foot-and-mouth disease, in Moser RL (ed): *Primary Care for Physician Assistants*. New York, McGraw-Hill, 1998, chap 2–15.]

2-26. **The correct answer is B.** Hand-foot-and-mouth disease is known for oral lesions in various stages that are gray to white in color with a red halo surrounding them. These will then ulcerate to shallow craters. These lesions are seen on the soft palate, uvula, and tonsillar areas but do not involve the buccal mucosa, lips, or tongue. [Sauls BL: Hand-foot-and-mouth disease, in Moser RL (ed): *Primary Care for Physician Assistants*. New York, McGraw-Hill, 1998, chap 2–15.]

2-27. **The correct answer is A.** Molluscum contagiosum is caused by a poxvirus. Herpes simplex causes herpes lesions of various types. Human papillomavirus causes condylomata acuminata (genital warts). Rotaviruses cause GI illness, and enterovirus causes various GI and dermatologic infections. [Sauls BL: Molluscum contagiosum, in Moser RL (ed): *Primary Care for Physician Assistants*. New York, McGraw-Hill, 1998, chap 2–22.]

2-28. **The correct answer is B.** HIV infection is known to be associated with multiple molluscum that may be up to five times the usual size. These are often found on the face and are most likely due to an immunocompromised status. The small papules found on an infant's face are called milia and disappear spontaneously. HPV causes genital warts or condylomata acuminata. Shaving may cause an irritant dermatitis, but not the umbilicated lesions of molluscum contagiosum. [Sauls BL: Molluscum contagiosum, in Moser RL (ed): *Primary Care for Physician Assistants*. New York, McGraw-Hill, 1998, chap 2–22.]

2-29. The correct answer is D. Molluscum contagiosum has few differential diagnoses. The two significant considerations are nodular basal cell carcinoma, which often has a central indentation, and keratoacanthoma, which is more like a crater. Both of these are rare in children, and children commonly get molluscum. Condylomata lata are flat, wartlike growths found on the perineal area in secondary syphilis, while condylomata acuminata are genital warts caused by human papillomavirus. Verruca vulgaris is common warts. [Sauls BL: Molluscum contagiosum, in Moser RL (ed): *Primary Care for Physician Assistants.* New York, McGraw-Hill, 1998, chap 2–22.]

2-30. The correct answer is A. Warts are more tender to lateral compression than to direct pressure. This is because the papilla of the wart contain nerves that are most sensitive to lateral compression. [Martin S: Common podiatric disorders, in Moser RL (ed): *Primary Care for Physician Assistants.* New York, McGraw-Hill, 1998, chap 2–10.]

2-31. The correct answer is D. Warts do not go beyond the epidermis and they do not have roots. Warts are caused by the human papillomavirus. Warts are frequently multiple and do not look like foreign-body reactions because warts have pinpoint bleeding, are tender to lateral compression, and do not have skin lines going through them. Foreign-body reactions usually have a singular puncture point evident. However, a puncture site from a foreign body may be invaded by the virus and become a verruca. [Martin S: Common podiatric disorders, in Moser RL (ed): *Primary Care for Physician Assistants.* New York, McGraw-Hill, 1998, chap 2–10.]

2-32. The correct answer is B. Cutting a V in the nail has never been proven to relieve pressure on the borders or distal edge. When patients try to dig out their own ingrown toenails, they frequently leave a spicule that further complicates the problem. Onychocryptosis can also occur on the distal edge when a nail that has been lost or removed is growing back. Antibiotics are usually not necessary to clear up a paronychia. Removal of the offending border and any associated granuloma followed by a soaking in warm water will usually alleviate the problem. However, if the patient is immune-compromised or the erythema extends proximal to the interphalangeal joint, antibiotics should be considered. [Martin S: Common podiatric disorders, in Moser RL (ed): *Primary Care for Physician Assistants.* New York, McGraw-Hill, 1998, chap 2–10.]

2-33. The correct answer is B. Bullous impetigo is caused by *Staphylococcus aureus,* which produces an exotoxin-inducing cleavage within the epidermis. [DiBaise M: Impetigo and ecthyma, in Moser RL (ed): *Primary Care for Physician Assistants.* New York, McGraw-Hill, 1998, chap 2–19.]

2-34. The correct answer is A. Mupirocin ointment (Bactroban) has been shown to be as effective as oral antibiotics in the treatment of impetigo. Penicillin and erythromycin are not appropriate due to potential resistance. Ciprofloxacin will not cover group A beta-hemolytic streptococci and 60 percent of methacillin-resistant *Staphylococcus aureus* (MRSA) infections are resistant to ciprofloxacin. [DiBaise M: Impetigo and ecthyma, in Moser RL (ed): *Primary Care for Physician Assistants.* New York, McGraw-Hill, 1998, chap 2–19.]

2-35. The correct answer is B. While the ASO titer rises in the presence of pharyngeal group A beta-hemolytic streptococci, it does not in impetigo. The remaining statements are true. [DiBaise M: Impetigo and ecthyma, in Moser RL (ed): *Primary Care for Physician Assistants.* New York, McGraw-Hill, 1998, chap 2–19.]

2-36. The correct answer is A. Lichen planus is in fact typically easy to diagnose, with its distinctive purple coloration (C), papular morphology (B), and involvement of the oral mucosa (D). Exceptions do occur; the hypertrophic variety of lichen planus seen on shins can mimic psoriasis. [Monroe J: Lichen planus, in Moser RL (ed): *Primary Care for Physician Assistants.* New York, McGraw-Hill, 1998, chap 2–20.]

2-37. **The correct answer is D.**   Lichen planus commonly appears as an infection in the mouth but only rarely occurs around the mouth. The other choices, planar (A), penile (B), and pruritic (C), are among the "P's" one is likely to see with lichen planus. The most constant of the "P's," and therefore the most useful, is "purple." [Monroe J: Lichen planus, in Moser RL (ed): *Primary Care for Physician Assistants*. New York, McGraw-Hill, 1998, chap 2–20.]

2-38. **The correct answer is E.**   All of the listed treatment options are acceptable. If the patient is symptomatic, palliative therapy with topical steroids or oral antihistamines is useful. UVB therapy can shorten the duration of the disease process if started within the first week of the eruption. [DiBaise M: Pityriasis rosea, in Moser RL (ed): *Primary Care for Physician Assistants*. New York, McGraw-Hill, 1998, chap 2–23.]

2-39. **The correct answer is D.**   A KOH can help in ruling out tinea corporis when only the herald patch is present. A skin biopsy is not necessary unless the generalized eruption does not resolve after 8 weeks. An RPR should be considered in all sexually active individuals, especially when there is an atypical presentation, such as palm and sole lesions. [DiBaise M: Pityriasis rosea, in Moser RL (ed): *Primary Care for Physician Assistants*. New York, McGraw-Hill, 1998, chap 2–23.]

2-40. **The correct answer is A.**   Tinea versicolor is the only tinea infection caused by a non-dermatophyte, *Pityrosporum*. The other tinea infections (pedis, corporis, capitis, cruris, unguium) are dermatophyte infections caused by organisms that favor the keratinized cells of skin, hair, and nails. [Sauls BL: Tinea infections of the skin, in Moser RL (ed): *Primary Care for Physician Assistants*. New York, McGraw-Hill, 1998, chap 2–28.]

2-41. **The correct answer is D.**   One of the most common sources of tinea pedis infection is the floors of athletic locker rooms and showers. Patients in this age group frequently get this infection from that source. The warm, moist environment promotes tinea growth. Dark socks tend to inhibit resolution of tinea infections, but do not cause them. *Rhus* contact causes a localized reaction of the skin known as rhus dermatitis or poison ivy, oak, and sumac. Symptoms include red skin, itching, and vesicle development. [Sauls BL: Tinea infections of the skin, in Moser RL (ed): *Primary Care for Physician Assistants*. New York, McGraw-Hill, 1998, chap 2–28.]

2-42. **The correct answer is D.**   The 10% KOH preparation or potassium hydroxide wet mount is a very simple, inexpensive office procedure that will assist in the diagnosis of tinea infections. Positive results include visualization of hyphae and/or buds upon microscopic examination. False-negative results are possible but it is difficult to get false-positive results unless the slide is misinterpreted. Fibers of cotton, thread, or hair are often mistaken for hyphae. Care must be taken to use clean slides and not to use a cotton swab to obtain the skin scraping. [Sauls BL: Tinea infections of the skin, in Moser RL (ed): *Primary Care for Physician Assistants*. New York, McGraw-Hill, 1998, chap 2–28.]

2-43. **The correct answer is C** and is important since it helps to distinguish scalp psoriasis from otherwise similar conditions such as tinea capitis or lichen planopilaris that do involve hair loss. As for A, scalp psoriasis can be quite difficult to treat, primarily because of the hair that blocks application of medication and penetration of light rays in PUVA treatment. It is also quite pruritic (B), which provokes scratching, which, in turn, provokes more scaling (the Koebner phenomenon). Finally, it is fairly common for scalp psoriasis to be the sole manifestation of that disease, so D is an incorrect statement. [Monroe J: Psoriasis, in Moser RL (ed): *Primary Care for Physician Assistants*. New York, McGraw-Hill, 1998, chap 2–24.]

2-44. The correct answer is B. Stopping the steroid for a while or switching to other agents (e.g., tar preparations or Dovonex) for a time can help combat tachyphylaxis. Woronoff's sign (A) is the term for the ring of hypopigmentation that sometimes surrounds the periphery of psoriasis plaques. Auspitz's sign (C) is the pinpoint bleeding that occurs when deep psoriatic scale is removed, for example, with a fingernail. It has been found to be nonspecific for psoriasis, but can be helpful in diagnosis. Munro's microabscesses (D) are pockets of neutrophils characteristically seen in histologic sections of psoriatic lesions, and are not related to treatment. [Monroe J: Psoriasis, in Moser RL (ed): *Primary Care for Physician Assistants.* New York, McGraw-Hill, 1998, chap 2–24.]

2-45. The correct answer is D. Precipitated sulfur is preferred, as the safety and efficacy of the other agents are not known, with the exception of lindane. Lindane should never be used in children under 2 years of age, or in pregnant or lactating women. [DiBaise M: Arthropod infestations, in Moser RL (ed): *Primary Care for Physician Assistants.* New York, McGraw-Hill, 1998, chap 2–5.]

2-46. The correct answer is B. Topical mupirocin is as effective as oral antibiotics for the treatment of secondary infections with *S. aureus* or group A beta-hemolytic streptococci. Pubic lice is one of the most contagious sexually transmitted diseases, but is not related to patient hygiene. Ivermectin is recommended only for treatment of crusted scabies in the immunocompromised patient. There are no reports in the literature of rheumatic fever occurring after secondary infection of the skin with group A beta-hemolytic streptococci. Acute glomerulonephritis has never followed an infection of *S. aureus*. It does occur after group A beta-hemolytic streptococci infection of the skin. [DiBaise M: Arthropod infestations, in Moser RL (ed): *Primary Care for Physician Assistants.* New York, McGraw-Hill, 1998, chap 2–5.]

2-47. The correct answer is C. Because of the potential for serious side effects, and ultimate worsening ("rebound") of atopic dermatitis, systemic corticosteroids are seldom used for atopic dermatitis. The other choices, antibiotics (A), frequent moisturization (B), and patient education (D), are commonly used. [Monroe J: Atopic dermatitis, in Moser RL (ed): *Primary Care for Physician Assistants.* New York, McGraw-Hill, 1998, chap 2–6.]

2-48. The correct answer is D. Bullous pemphigoid is in fact characterized by symmetrical involvement of limbs. Choice A is incorrect since bullous pemphigoid is often anything but benign in its clinical course. It is characterized by a negative Nikolsky's sign, so B is incorrect. The latter means that the blisters of bullous pemphigoid are tense and not at all easily ruptured, so C is incorrect. [Monroe J: Bullous blistering diseases, in Moser RL (ed): *Primary Care for Physician Assistants.* New York, McGraw-Hill, 1998, chap 2–8.]

2-49. The correct answer is A, molluscum contagiosum, since it presents with firm papules and not with blisters of any kind. All the other choices (lichen planus, insect bites, and pityriasis rosea) can and do present as bullous processes. [Monroe J: Bullous blistering diseases, in Moser RL (ed): *Primary Care for Physician Assistants.* New York, McGraw-Hill, 1998, chap 2–8.]

2-50. The correct answer is D. It is caused by the bacterial organism *Erysipelothrix rhusiopathiae* and is characterized by an indolent coarse and relatively asymptomatic lesion most typically found on the hands and fingers. Necrotizing fasciitis (A), by contrast, is rapidly evolving and the patient is highly symptomatic. Cryptococcal cellulitis (B) is found almost exclusively in the seriously immunocompromised patient. Erysipelas (C) is, likewise, rapidly evolving, affecting mostly the face. [Monroe J: Cellulitis, in Moser RL (ed): *Primary Care for Physician Assistants.* New York, McGraw-Hill, 1998, chap 2–9.]

2-51. The correct answer is A.   The oleoresin of the rhus plants (poison ivy, oak, and sumac) is the black dots found on the backs of the plant leaves. Contact with this resin causes an inflammatory reaction of the skin in sensitive individuals. The fluid found in the vesicles of persons with rhus dermatitis contains serous fluid, not the allergen. English ivy plants are not members of the rhus family, do not have oleoresin on the undersides of their leaves, and do not cause rhus dermatitis. Insects do not carry the rhus allergen in their saliva. [Sauls BL: Contact dermatitis, in Moser RL (ed): *Primary Care for Physician Assistants*. New York, McGraw-Hill, 1998, chap 2–1.]

2-52. The correct answer is D.   Nickel is commonly a component of an alloy used to make cheaper jewelry as well as buckles and snaps. Individuals often develop a contact dermatitis from contact with this alloy. The alloy also contains chromium and it is unproved exactly which of the two is the actual cause of the reaction. Silver and gold are also used to make jewelry. Neither of these causes contact dermatitis reactions. Gold causes skin reactions only when used systemically, as in IM gold injections for rheumatoid arthritis. [Sauls BL: Contact dermatitis, in Moser RL (ed): *Primary Care for Physician Assistants*. New York, McGraw-Hill, 1998, chap 2–1.]

2-53. The correct answer is B.   The cardinal rule when choosing a dressing is to keep the ulcer tissue moist to promote healing, and the surrounding tissue dry. If the surrounding tissue is kept moist this may increase skin breakdown in this area. A dressing that adheres to the wound will remove both vital and nonvital tissue, and actually damages the wound. [United States Department of Health and Human Services, Agency for Health Care Policy and Research: Pressure ulcers in adults: Treatment of pressure ulcers. *Clinical Practice Guidelines* No 15, 1994; Segal-Gidan F: Decubitus ulcers, in Moser RL (ed): *Primary Care for Physician Assistants*. New York, McGraw-Hill, 1998, chap 2–11.]

2-54. The correct answer is D, since HSV infections are the most common triggers for erythema multiforme minor. Therefore, one of the very first questions in the history taking should be about a possible recent HSV episode. Lots of other potential triggers for erythema multiforme have been suggested, including stress (A), excessive sun exposure (B), and exposure to animals (C), but these are unsubstantiated anecdotal reports. Interestingly, some feel that these can be triggers for erythema multiforme, but only because they can trigger herpes. [Monroe J: Erythema multiforme, in Moser RL (ed): *Primary Care for Physician Assistants*. New York, McGraw-Hill, 1998, chap 2–12.]

2-55. The correct answer is B because of the three most common causes of erythema nodosum in this country, the most common is the oral contraceptive. The other two most common causes are *Streptococcal* infection and sarcoidosis. Stress has been postulated, but not documented, as a possible cause of erythema nodosum, so A is not the best choice. Certainly one can travel to foreign countries and fall prey to unusual or rare diseases capable of triggering erythema nodosum, such as leprosy, but one would want to rule out more common causes first, so C is not the best choice. Patients very often present with "insect bites" as a self-diagnosis, but erythema nodosum is characterized by the *lack* of epidermal changes (bite site, scabbing, or other central break in the skin) one would expect to see with insect bites, so D is not the best choice. [Monroe J: Erythema nodosum, in Moser RL (ed): *Primary Care for Physician Assistants*. New York, McGraw-Hill, 1998, chap 2–13.]

2-56. The correct answer is C.   The bilateral hilar adenopathy often found on the chest x-rays of erythema nodosum patients is usually a common, benign finding of unknown origin, and frequently clears in a week or two. Malignancies, such as lymphoma (A), have been implicated as a cause of erythema nodosum, but are much less likely to cause the radiological findings. Even though these radiological findings certainly suggest sarcoidosis, the chest x-ray should be repeated before that diagnosis is seriously entertained, so B is an incorrect choice. It is a classic mistake in working up erythema nodosum to settle on sarcoidosis too early. Tuberculosis can trigger erythema nodosum but is unlikely to be manifested by these particular x-ray findings. TB is much more likely to involve the apices of the lungs, so D is an incorrect choice. [Monroe J: Erythema nodosum, in Moser RL (ed): *Primary Care for Physician Assistants*. New York, McGraw-Hill, 1998, chap 2–13.]

2-57.   The correct answer is C.   Assuming there is an identifiable trigger, finding and eliminating this underlying cause of erythema nodosum are essential. Proper treatment of erythema nodosum includes bed rest, NSAIDS for symptomatic use, or oral potassium iodide. However, finding and eliminating the underlying cause are very basic tenets of treating erythema nodosum. Broad-spectrum antibiotics (A) seldom have a place in treatment of erythema nodosum unless the underlying cause requires them. Topical steroids (B) are of no use in erythema nodosum because the disease process is well below the surface and thus out of reach of these agents. The use of systemic steroids (D) is seldom necessary, and is indicated only in severe cases where ordinary treatment has failed and when infectious causation has been ruled out, since steroids have the potential to lessen the body's immune response to infection. [Monroe J: Erythema nodosum, in Moser RL (ed): *Primary Care for Physician Assistants*. New York, McGraw-Hill, 1998, chap 2–13.]

2-58.   The correct answer is D.   The lip is one of the more common areas involved in angioedema, but many others have been reported, including palms and soles, where it tends to be slightly tender to touch. Whatever the location, angioedema usually resolves within 48 h, if not much sooner. Cellulitis (A) is commonly misdiagnosed, and is incorrect in this case, since it, unlike angioedema, would be red, hot, and tender, and would probably not resolve within 48 h, even with treatment. Hereditary angioedema (HAE) (B) does present with angioedema, but is rare, so is not the likely diagnosis. However, possible family history of unexplained respiratory distress needs to be investigated to help rule out HAE. Unlike angioedema, contact dermatitis (C) would present as an epidermal (surface) papulovesicular (small bumps and blisters), highly pruritic process that would take days to weeks to resolve, so it is incorrect. Interestingly, urticaria/angioedema can be triggered by contact with substances previously sensitized to, such as plants and animal dander. [Monroe J: Urticaria, in Moser RL (ed): *Primary Care for Physician Assistants*. New York, McGraw-Hill, 1998, chap 2–2.]

2-59.   The correct answer is A.   Even though systemic antibiotics are quite commonly prescribed, they are in fact seldom necessary if the other measures, hot compresses (B), incision and drainage (C), and elimination of known etiologic factors (D), are taken. There are exceptions that include furunculosis in immunocompromised patients, in patients with systemic symptomatology, or in severe cases unresponsive to conservative treatment. [Monroe J: Folliculitis, in Moser RL (ed): *Primary Care for Physician Assistants*. New York, McGraw-Hill, 1998, chap 2–14.]

2-60.   The correct answer is A.   Seldom does this problem require any treatment at all, and usually lasts about a week, exceptions being the immunocompromised or symptomatic patient, so B is incorrect, as is D. Healthy doses of reassurance are in order. In some states reporting of this problem to local health authorities is mandatory, and it is always a good idea since families thus afflicted will be anxious to get the facts on how to prevent recurrences (proper filtration, chemical water treatment, temperature, limitation of fecal contaminants). Incising and draining each pustule (D) is not necessary, though culture and sensitivity of pustular material are sometimes necessary to establish the diagnosis. This problem is not at all contagious, so C is an incorrect choice. Interestingly, it is not at all uncommon to have just as many people *un*affected by this as those who were, even though they were all in the tub at the same time. [Monroe J: Folliculitis, in Moser RL (ed): *Primary Care for Physician Assistants*. New York, McGraw-Hill, 1998, chap 2–14.]

SECTION 3
EAR, NOSE, AND THROAT

3. EAR, NOSE, AND THROAT

QUESTIONS

DIRECTIONS: Each question below contains suggested responses. Choose the **one best** response to each question.

3-1. Which of the following is NOT a sign or symptom of allergic rhinitis?

(A) pale, boggy nasal mucosa
(B) clear discharge
(C) vesicular lesions of the oral mucosa
(D) cough
(E) fatigue

3-2. Which of the following is NOT utilized in the treatment of allergic rhinitis?

(A) cromolyn
(B) terbutaline
(C) terfenadine
(D) corticosteriods
(E) allergen avoidance

3-3. What distinguishes allergic rhinitis from vasomotor rhinitis?

(A) nasal congestion is a symptom of only allergic rhinitis
(B) vasomotor rhinitis symptoms include sneezing
(C) mast cell histamine release occurs in vasomotor rhinitis
(D) vasomotor rhinitis does not involve a parasympathetic reflex
(E) vasomotor rhinitis is an allergen-mediated variation of allergic rhinitis

3-4. Which of the following is a common allergen in perennial allergic rhinitis?

(A) ragweed
(B) food
(C) tree pollens
(D) grass pollens
(E) dust mites

3-5. Expected symptoms of laryngitis include all of the following EXCEPT

(A) hoarseness
(B) dysphonia
(C) hemoptysis
(D) cough
(E) ear pain

3-6. A patient with acute onset of hoarseness complains that there has been no improvement after 4 weeks of conservative treatment. He had no gastrointestinal pain, throat pain, fever, cough, or upper respiratory symptoms initially. He has been resting his voice but continues to smoke. Your next step in treatment should include

(A) referral to an otolaryngologist
(B) antibiotics
(C) continued conservative treatment
(D) speech therapy
(E) a trial of H2 antagonist

3-7. Laryngitis caused by voice abuse (yelling, overuse, inappropriate phonation) may be due to which of the following?

(A) laryngeal polyps
(B) vocal nodules
(C) laryngeal cancer
(D) vocal cord paralysis
(E) A and B only

3-8. Benign causes of hoarseness include which of the following?

(A) hyperkeratosis
(B) laryngeal polyps
(C) leukoplakia
(D) vocal cord paralysis
(E) B and D only

3-9. The MOST common predisposing risk factor for otitis media in children is

(A) allergies
(B) day-care attendance
(C) adenoidal hypertrophy
(D) upper respiratory infections
(E) tonsillar hypertrophy

3-10. The MOST common biological cause of spontaneous rupture of the tympanic membrane in children is

(A) beta lactamase–producing strains of *Haemophilus influenzae*
(B) *Moraxella (Branhamella) catarrhalis*
(C) group A beta-hemolytic *Streptococcus*
(D) respiratory syncytial viruses
(E) *Pseudomonas aeruginosa*

3-11. In the physical assessment of a child with possible otitis media, the MOST predictive sign is

(A) decreased motility of the tympanic membrane
(B) the presence of pus in the ear canal
(C) tragal tenderness
(D) fever
(E) redness of the tympanic membrane

3-12. Which of the following pathogens is NOT a common etiologic agent for mastoiditis?

(A) *Haemophilus influenzae*
(B) *Moraxella catarrhalis*
(C) *Pseudomonas aeruginosa*
(D) *Streptococcus pneumoniae*

3-13. Which of the following symptoms is generally seen in mastoiditis but NOT in otitis media?

(A) otalgia
(B) fever
(C) postauricular pain
(D) all of the above

3-14. Which of the following could be considered as an extracranial complication of mastoiditis?

(A) labyrinthitis
(B) meningitis
(C) brain abscess
(D) all of the above

3-15. Which of the following is NOT appropriate first-line therapy for acute mastoiditis?

(A) cefixime (Suprax)
(B) azithromycin (Zithromax)
(C) amoxicillin/clavulanic potassium (Augmentin)
(D) cefuroxime axetil (Ceftin)

3-16. What is the MOST common radiographic feature seen in mastoiditis?

(A) air-fluid levels
(B) loss of mastoid air cells
(C) marked soft tissue swelling
(D) all of the above

3-17. The paranasal sinuses MOST commonly infected are

(A) sphenoid
(B) maxillary
(C) ethmoid
(D) frontal

3-18. The MOST common etiology of bacterial sinusitis is

(A) *Streptococcus pneumoniae*
(B) *Staphylococcus aureus*
(C) *Moraxella catarrhalis*
(D) group A beta-hemolytic *Streptococcus*

3-19. The paranasal sinuses MOST prone to osteomyelitis are

(A) sphenoid
(B) maxillary
(C) ethmoid
(D) frontal

3-20. The following are complications of sinusitis EXCEPT

(A) meningitis
(B) periorbital cellulitis
(C) peritonsillar abscess
(D) osteomyelitis

3-21. The MOST common complication of acute bacterial sinusitis is

(A) chronic sinusitis
(B) osteomyelitis
(C) cellulitis
(D) cavernous sinus thrombosis

3-22. The classic triad of clinical manifestations associated with infectious mononucleosis is

(A) fever, malaise, and pharyngitis
(B) cervical adenopathy, splenomegaly, and pharyngitis
(C) fever, lymphadenopathy, and pharyngitis
(D) malaise, cervical adenopathy, and pharyngitis
(E) fever, pharyngitis, and splenomegaly

3-23. A 15-year-old female high school student presents to the outpatient clinic complaining of severe sore throat and malaise for 3 days. Physical examination reveals a fever of 39°C (102°F), palatal petechia, and posterior cervical adenopathy. Tonsils are enlarged with exudate. Spleen and liver are not enlarged or tender. Expected laboratory findings in this patient include which of the following?

(A) lymphocytosis
(B) decreased liver enzymes
(C) positive heterophile antibody test (monospot test)
(D) all of the above
(E) A and C only

3-24. Management of infectious mononucleosis includes

(A) instructing the patient to avoid contact sports or strenuous exercise
(B) rest during the acute phase and gradual return to normal activity
(C) symptomatic treatment of fever and pharyngitis
(D) penicillin or erythromycin for treatment of bacterial pharyngitis
(E) all of the above

3-25. Complications of infectious mononucleosis include

(A) hematologic
(B) neurologic
(C) hepatic
(D) cardiac
(E) all of the above

3. EAR, NOSE, AND THROAT

ANSWERS

3-1. **The correct answer is C.** Vesicular mucosal lesions are not characteristic of allergic rhinitis. On examination, a pale, boggy nasal mucosa is common. A clear nasal discharge with cough is a common sign of allergic rhinitis. Fatigue, although nonspecific, could also be present. [Dehn R: Allergic rhinitis, in Moser RL (ed): *Primary Care for Physician Assistants*. New York, McGraw-Hill, 1998, chap 3–4.]

3-2. **The correct answer is B.** Terbutaline is used in the management of asthma, not allergic rhinitis. The other choices are all used in treating allergic rhinitis. [Dehn R: Allergic rhinitis, in Moser RL (ed): *Primary Care for Physician Assistants*. New York, McGraw-Hill, 1998, chap 3–4.]

3-3. **The correct answer is D.** Vasomotor rhinitis does involve a parasympathetic reflex. [Dehn R: Allergic rhinitis, in Moser RL (ed): *Primary Care for Physician Assistants*. New York, McGraw-Hill, 1998, chap 3–4.]

3-4. **The correct answer is E.** Dust mites, present year-round in the environment, are the most common allergen involved in perennial allergic rhinitis on the list. All other choices are common seasonal allergens. [Dehn R: Allergic rhinitis, in Moser RL (ed): *Primary Care for Physician Assistants*. New York, McGraw-Hill, 1998, chap 3–4.]

3-5. **The correct answer is C.** Symptoms of laryngitis include hoarseness, dysphonia, irritating cough, and throat or ear pain. Hemoptysis is rare. [Warnimont S: Laryngitis, in Moser RL (ed): *Primary Care for Physician Assistants*. New York, McGraw-Hill, 1998, chap 3–6; Rakel R: *Saunders Manual of Medical Practice*. Philadelphia, Saunders, 1996, p 108.]

3-6. **The correct answer is A.** A patient with persistent hoarseness that does not respond to conservative therapy should be referred to an otolaryngologist for direct laryngoscopy and biopsy. Most patients with acute laryngitis recover in 2 to 3 weeks. Antibiotics may be useful in selected patients when fever, pain, productive cough, or purulent sputum suggest bacterial infection. Speech therapy is useful for persons who abuse their voices chronically. Gastroesophageal reflux can cause laryngitis. Initial history should include questions about GI symptoms. [Warnimont S: Laryngitis, in Moser RL (ed): *Primary Care for Physician Assistants*. New York, McGraw-Hill, 1998, chap 3–6; Rakel R: *Saunders Manual of Medical Practice*. Philadelphia, Saunders, 1996, p 109.]

3-7. **The correct answer is E.** Laryngeal polyps, vocal nodules, contact ulcers, hyperkeratosis, and leukoplakia can all be the result of voice abuse. Carcinoma and vocal cord paralysis both cause hoarseness but are not directly caused by voice abuse. [Warnimont S: Laryngitis, in Moser RL (ed): *Primary Care for Physician Assistants*. New York, McGraw-Hill, 1998, chap 3–6; Curtis LC: Common ear, nose, and throat problems. *Phys Assist* 14(10): 21–22, 1990.]

3-8. **The correct answer is E.** Laryngeal polyps, vocal nodules, contact ulcers, and vocal cord paralysis are all nonmalignant causes of hoarseness. Premalignant causes include hyperkeratosis and leukoplakia. Premalignant and other suspicious lesions of the vocal cords should be biopsied. [Warnimont S: Laryngitis, in Moser RL (ed): *Primary Care for*

Physician Assistants. New York, McGraw-Hill, 1998, chap 3–6; Curtis LC: Common ear, nose, and throat problems. *Phys Assist* 14(10): 21–22, 1990.]

3-9. The correct answer is D. Children average 6 to 9 upper respiratory infections per year during the first 6 years of life. Upper respiratory infections are the most common predisposing factor, followed closely by day-care attendance. Allergies and adenoidal hypertrophy are less common factors. Tonsillar hypertrophy has little or no relationship to otitis-prone children. [Moser RL: Otitis media, in Moser RL (ed): *Primary Care for Physician Assistants.* New York, McGraw-Hill, 1998, chap 3–2.]

3-10. The correct answer is C. Although spontaneous rupture can occur with any ear infection, regardless of the pathogen, group A beta-hemolytic *Streptococcus* (GABHS) has been found to be the most common. Selecting an appropriate antibiotic that covers GABHS would be important if a spontaneous perforation is present. *Pseudomonas aeruginosa* may be present in otitis externa, and is a rare middle-ear pathogen. [Moser RL: Otitis media, in Moser RL (ed): *Primary Care for Physician Assistants.* New York, McGraw-Hill, 1998, chap 3–2.]

3-11. The correct answer is A. Decreased motility of the tympanic membrane (TM), assessed by the pneumatic otoscope, has been found to be more predictive than color changes in diagnosing acute otitis media. Crying and fever can cause the TM to appear red. Acute infections may also have an opacified, yellow appearance without redness. Tragal tenderness is a sign commonly seen in otitis externa, not otitis media. The presence of pus in the ear canal is nonspecific, and is not predictive of a middle-ear source. [Moser RL: Otitis media, in Moser RL (ed): *Primary Care for Physician Assistants.* New York, McGraw-Hill, 1998, chap 3–2.]

3-12. The correct answer is C. Mastoiditis is most frequently caused by the same organisms that cause otitis media, *Haemophilus influenzae, Moraxella catarrhalis,* and *Streptococcus pneumoniae.* Although *Pseudomonas aeruginosa* is frequently implicated in otitis externa, it rarely produces an inner-ear infection. [Scott PM: Mastoiditis, in Moser RL (ed): *Primary Care for Physician Assistants.* New York, McGraw-Hill, 1998, chap 3–12.]

3-13. The correct answer is C. Otalgia and fever are common symptoms in both mastoiditis and otitis media. [Scott PM: Mastoiditis, in Moser RL (ed): *Primary Care for Physician Assistants.* New York, McGraw-Hill, 1998, chap 3–12.]

3-14. The correct answer is A. Although meningitis and brain abscess are both potential complications of mastoiditis, they are intracranial, not extracranial. Labyrinthitis is the only extracranial complication listed. [Scott PM: Mastoiditis, in Moser RL (ed): *Primary Care for Physician Assistants.* New York, McGraw-Hill, 1998, chap 3–12.]

3-15. The correct answer is B. Although azithromycin is probably effective against the most common pathogens causing mastoiditis, it is not usually used as a first-line choice. [Scott PM: Mastoiditis, in Moser RL (ed): *Primary Care for Physician Assistants.* New York, McGraw-Hill, 1998, chap 3–12.]

3-16. The correct answer is B. The most common radiographic feature of mastoiditis is cloudiness of the mastoid air cells or frank loss of the air cells by the destruction of the bony partitions between them. Soft tissue swelling could be seen. However, unless there was an associated abscess, it is generally mild. Air-fluid levels are rare in mastoiditis. [Scott PM: Mastoiditis, in Moser RL (ed): *Primary Care for Physician Assistants.* New York, McGraw-Hill, 1998, chap 3–12.]

3-17. The correct answer is B. The maxillary sinus, the largest and the lowest (anatomically), is the most common sinus that becomes infected. [Hansen M: Sinusitis, in Moser RL (ed): *Primary Care for Physician Assistants.* New York, McGraw-Hill, 1998, chap 3–1.]

3-18. **The correct answer is A.** Although all of the responses can cause sinusitis, *S. pneumoniae* is by far the most common bacterial etiology. [Hansen M: Sinusitis, in Moser RL (ed): *Primary Care for Physician Assistants.* New York, McGraw-Hill, 1998, chap 3–1.]

3-19. **The correct answer is D.** The frontal sinuses statistically are the ones most commonly prone to osteomyelitis. [Hansen M: Sinusitis, in Moser RL (ed): *Primary Care for Physician Assistants.* New York, McGraw-Hill, 1998, chap 3–1.]

3-20. **The correct answer is C.** Peritonsillar abscesses are not associated with sinusitis in most cases. Sinusitis can result in meningitis, periorbital cellulitis, and osteomyelitis. [Hansen M: Sinusitis, in Moser RL (ed): *Primary Care for Physician Assistants.* New York, McGraw-Hill, 1998, chap 3–1.]

3-21. **The correct answer is A.** The most common complication is chronicity. The other choices are rare and serious complications. [Hansen M: Sinusitis, in Moser RL (ed): *Primary Care for Physician Assistants.* New York, McGraw-Hill, 1998, chap 3–1.]

3-22. **The correct answer is C.** Infectious mononucleosis classically presents with fever, lymphadenopathy, and pharyngitis. Fever and posterior and/or anterior cervical adenopathy occur in 90 percent of patients. Severe pharyngitis most often prompts patients to seek medical treatment. Patients also complain of headache and malaise. Periorbital edema, palatal petechia, hepatomegaly, splenomegaly, and rash may be seen on physical examination. [Cohen JI: Epstein-Barr virus infections, including infectious mononucleosis, in Fauci AS, Braunwald E, Isselbacher KJ, et al (eds): *Harrison's Principles of Internal Medicine*, 14th ed. New York, McGraw-Hill, 1998, p 1089.]

3-23. **The correct answer is E.** Laboratory tests for mononucleosis will reveal mild hepatitis manifested by elevated liver transaminases and modest leukocytosis with most of the increase in lymphocytes. Mild neutropenia and thrombocytopenia are also seen. The presence of heterophile antibodies (found in 90 to 95 percent of adolescents with mononucleosis) is confirmed by the monospot test. [Cohen JI: Epstein-Barr virus infections, including infectious mononucleosis, in Fauci AS, Braunwald E, Isselbacher KJ, et al (eds): *Harrison's Principles of Internal Medicine*, 14th ed. New York, McGraw-Hill, 1998, p 1090.]

3-24. **The correct answer is E.** Treatment of uncomplicated infectious mononucleosis is supportive. Warm saline gargle or topical anesthetic will relieve sore throat. Acetaminophen is used for fever. Superinfection by group A beta-hemolytic *Streptococcus* will require treatment with penicillin or erythromycin. Amoxicillin or ampicillin should be avoided since they will cause a rash in persons with mononucleosis. Splenomegaly is seen in 50 percent of patients. Strenuous activity or contact sports increase risk of rupture of the enlarged spleen. (Rakel R: *Saunders Manual of Medical Practice.* Philadelphia, Saunders, 1996, p 873.)

3-25. **The correct answer is E.** Complications of infectious mononucleosis are rare but may be the major manifestation of the illness. Hematologic complications include hemolytic anemia, mild thrombocytopenia in 50 percent of cases, and mild granulocytopenia. Severe hematologic complications can occur. Splenic rupture is rare. It is accompanied by abdominal pain and occurs in the second or third week of illness. Neurologic complications may be the presenting manifestation of the illness. Most frequent are cranial nerve palsies (especially Bell's palsy) and encephalitis. The majority of patients with neurologic complications recover spontaneously. Hepatitis is common. Almost 90 percent of patients will have elevated serum transaminases. Cardiac complications are uncommon but can occur. Airway obstruction can occur from adenopathy. Pulmonary infiltrates may occur, especially in children. [Cohen JI: Epstein-Barr virus infections, including infectious mononucleosis, in Fauci AS, Braunwald E, Isselbacher KJ, et al (eds): *Harrison's Principles of Internal Medicine*, 14th ed. New York, McGraw-Hill, 1998, p 1090.]

SECTION 4
EMERGENCY MEDICINE

4. EMERGENCY MEDICINE

QUESTIONS

DIRECTIONS: Each question below contains suggested responses. Choose the **one best** response to each question.

4-1. Traditionally, the bacteria MOST closely associated with epiglottitis is

(A) *Haemophilus influenzae*
(B) *Streptococcus pyogenes*
(C) *Candida albicans*
(D) herpes simplex

4-2. The primary management in epiglottitis is

(A) hemodynamic
(B) airway
(C) antimicrobial
(D) all of the above

4-3. The SINGLE factor MOST closely associated with a decreased occurrence of epiglottitis is

(A) epiglottitis protocols
(B) early intervention with nasotracheal intubation
(C) administration of the Hib vaccine
(D) early administration of ceftriaxone sodium (Rocephin)
(E) none of the above

4-4. A lateral soft tissue neck film finding consistent with epiglottitis is

(A) epiglottic width greater than 8 mm
(B) aryepiglottic folds larger than 7 mm
(C) decrease in the angle of the valleculae
(D) an increase in the ratio of the hypopharyngeal to tracheal air column width
(E) all of the above

4-5. The clinical feature of shock that is BEST explained by inadequate cellular oxygen delivery is

(A) cool, cyanotic extremities
(B) hypotension
(C) bradycardia
(D) hyperglycemia
(E) metabolic acidosis

4-6. In a patient in shock, found to have tachycardia, tachypnea, jugular venous distention, a tympanic left hemithorax, hypotension, and no apical breath sounds over the left lung, the PRIMARY diagnostic consideration is

(A) a massive pulmonary embolism
(B) a myocardial infarction
(C) a gram-negative septic state
(D) a tension pneumothorax
(E) a pericardial effusion

4-7. The therapy for shock that would NOT directly affect tissue perfusion is

(A) vasopressors (dopamine and similar pharmacologic agents)
(B) fluid resuscitation (intravenous fluid replacement)
(C) albumin administration
(D) application of pneumatic antishock garments
(E) oxygen

4-8. Which of the following overdoses would cause miosis (constricted pupils)?

(A) hallucinogens
(B) marijuana
(C) amphetamines
(D) narcotics
(E) ethanol

4-9. Which of the following overdoses is NOT correctly paired with its antidote?

(A) acetaminophen: *N*-acetylcysteine (Mucomyst)
(B) morphine: naloxone (Narcan)
(C) iron: deferoxamine mesylate
(D) benzodiazepines: flumazenil (Romazicon)
(E) lithium: charcoal

4-10. In heroin overdose you would expect to see all of the following EXCEPT

(A) miotic pupils
(B) increased respiration
(C) decreased gastrointestinal motility
(D) bradycardia
(E) hypotension

4-11. Emesis is indicated in which of the following?

(A) 2-month-old infant
(B) unconscious patient
(C) hydrocarbon ingestion
(D) strong acid or alkali
(E) aspirin overdose

4-12. Which one of the following is NOT correctly paired with its associated injury?

(A) acetaminophen: hepatotoxicity
(B) isopropyl alcohol: hemorrhagic gastritis
(C) methanol: blindness
(D) tricyclic
    antidepressants: cardiac
(E) cocaine: renal toxicity

4-13. All but which of the following would you expect to see in *severe* hypothermia?

(A) shivering
(B) hypotension
(C) cardiac arrhythmias
(D) altered mental status
(E) neurologic abnormalities

4-14. Which of the following leads to an increased risk for developing hypothermia?

(A) mental impairment
(B) extremes in age (very young/very old)
(C) intoxication
(D) endocrine abnormalities
(E) all of the above

4-15. Anhidrosis in heat stroke is

(A) rare among well-conditioned athletes
(B) seen in classic heat stroke only
(C) common in exertional heat stroke
(D) absent in up to 50 percent of the cases of exertional heat stroke

4-16. Which set of conditions should be considered in the differential diagnosis of heat stroke?

(A) CNS infection, salicylate overdose, TB, malaria
(B) encephalitis, cerebral falciparum malaria, dehydration, Alzheimer's disease
(C) thyroid storm, adrenal failure, haloperidol therapy, meningitis
(D) CNS infection, cocaine overdose, pheochromo-cytoma, neuroleptic malignant syndrome
(E) myoglobinuria, dyskinesia, malaria, anticholinergic overdose

4-17. What is the MAIN objective of a fluid challenge?

(A) activate antidiuretic hormone
(B) avoid gastrointestinal irritation
(C) encourage diuresis
(D) maintain effective circulatory volume

4-18. Which of the following fluids offers the GREATEST expansion of the extracellular fluid?

(A) albumin
(B) 5% dextrose in water
(C) normal saline
(D) packed red blood cells

4-19. One liter of normal saline will expand the extracellular fluid volume by

(A) 1%
(B) 2%
(C) 6%
(D) 10%
(E) 50%

4-20. Tears are lost at __% dehydration.

(A) 5%
(B) 7%
(C) 10%
(D) 12%
(E) 15%

4-21. In hyponatremic states, total body water is

(A) increased
(B) normal
(C) reduced
(D) all of the above are possible

4-22. Low-fluid-volume states

(A) inhibit ADH
(B) inhibit the renin-angiotensin system
(C) produce bradycardia
(D) stimulate sodium retention
(E) sustain effective circulatory volume

4-23. Which of the following is NOT seen in hyponatremia?

(A) confusion
(B) lethargy
(C) muscle twitching
(D) paralysis
(E) seizure activity

4-24. Acidosis

(A) enhances bicarbonate excretion
(B) inhibits bicarbonate regeneration
(C) inhibits hydrogen secretion
(D) inhibits respirations
(E) stimulates excretion of ammonium

4-25. Match the following conditions with the most likely acid-base disorder. (Each answer may be used once, more than once, or not at all.)

___ anxiety   (A) metabolic acidosis
___ COPD   (B) metabolic alkalosis
___ hyperventilation   (C) respiratory acidosis
___ milk-alkali syndrome (D) respiratory alkalosis
___ salicylate ingestion

4-26. In acute diabetic ketoacidosis, serum potassium is MOST commonly measured as

(A) absent
(B) bound
(C) increased
(D) reduced

4-27. Which of the following conditions would cause a high anion gap?

(A) excess albumin
(B) excess bicarbonate
(C) excess chloride
(D) reduced phosphate
(E) reduced sodium

4-28. Which of the following types of animals inflicts the GREATEST number of bite injuries per year in the United States?

(A) cats
(B) humans
(C) dogs
(D) snakes

4-29. An infected cat bite will MOST likely have which ONE of the following as the infectious organism?

(A) *Streptococcus* species
(B) *Bacteroides fragilis*
(C) *Eikenella corrodens*
(D) *Pasteurella multocida*

4-30. Which of the following pharmacologic agents should be used in the treatment of cat bites?

(A) erythromycin
(B) amoxicillin-clavulanate
(C) penicillin
(D) cephalexin

4. EMERGENCY MEDICINE

ANSWERS

4-1. The correct answer is A. Prior to 1990, *Haemophilus influenzae* type b was the most common organism, accounting for 80 to 90 percent of the disease. The other organisms listed, *Streptococcus pneumoniae, Candida albicans*, and herpes simplex have all been increasingly documented as the causative agent since the administration of the Hib vaccine. [Kroenke N: Epiglottitis: Acute supraglottic laryngitis, in Moser RL (ed): *Primary Care for Physician Assistants*. New York, McGraw-Hill, 1998, chap 4–5.]

4-2. The correct answer is B. Airway management remains the foremost goal of the treatment of any patient with epiglottitis. Airway management is key, whether it is through immediate emergency intervention with intubation or through delayed observation and operative intervention. [Kroenke N: Epiglottitis: Acute supraglottic laryngitis, in Moser RL (ed): *Primary Care for Physician Assistants*. New York, McGraw-Hill, 1998, chap 4–5.]

4-3. The correct answer is C. Administration of the Hib vaccine has led to a decreased incidence of epiglottitis. *Haemophilus influenzae* now only accounts for about 25 percent of the disease's occurrences. Epiglottitis protocols are recommended to assure adequate mobilization of necessary staff to appropriately treat the patient. Administration of antibiotics should take place only after airway stabilization. [Kroenke N: Epiglottitis: Acute supraglottic laryngitis, in Moser RL (ed): *Primary Care for Physician Assistants*. New York, McGraw-Hill, 1998, chap 4–5.]

4-4. The correct answer is E. Neck films are more accurate when taken during inspiration and with the neck slightly extended. Radiographs may be taken portably or with provider escort. Epiglottic width greater than 8 mm, aryepiglottic folds larger than 7 mm, a decrease in the angle of the valleculae, and an increase in the ratio of the hypopharyngeal to tracheal air column width together are indicative of epiglottitis. [Kroenke N: Epiglottitis: Acute supraglottic laryngitis, in Moser RL (ed): *Primary Care for Physician Assistants*. New York, McGraw-Hill, 1998, chap 4–5.]

4-5. The correct answer is E. Secondary to inadequate cellular oxygenation, cellular metabolism shifts to anaerobic pathways. The resultant lactic acid and other metabolic by-products induce a metabolic acidotic state. [Sefcik DJ: Shock, in Moser RL (ed): *Primary Care for Physician Assistants*. New York, McGraw-Hill, 1998, chap 4–7.]

4-6. The correct answer is D. With a tension pneumothorax, the clinician would expect to be unable to auscultate breath sounds over the apex of the involved hemithorax, or find tympany on the ipsilateral side of the pneumothorax, or discover signs of impeded right heart filling (i.e., jugular venous distention), along with nonspecific signs of shock, such as hypotension, tachycardia, and tachypnea. A massive pulmonary embolism, a myocardial infarction, gram-negative sepsis, and a pericardial effusion would not demonstrate tympany or absent breath sounds. [Sefcik DJ: Shock, in Moser RL (ed): *Primary Care for Physician Assistants*. New York, McGraw-Hill, 1998, chap 4–7.]

4-7. The correct answer is E. Although oxygen administration is generally employed in the management of shock, its effectiveness is directed toward improving tissue oxygenation. Factors that affect the cardiac output or total peripheral vascular resistance, such as vasopressors, intravenous fluids, albumin administration, and the application of pneumatic antishock garments, would be expected to improve tissue perfusion. [Sefcik DJ: Shock, in Moser RL (ed): *Primary Care for Physician Assistants*. New York, McGraw-Hill, 1998, chap 4–7.]

4-8. The correct answer is D. Hallucinogens, marijuana, and amphetamines produce a mydriatic pupillary response (dilated pupils), while ethanol is not generally associated with pupillary changes. [Newell KA: Poisoning and overdose, in Moser RL (ed): *Primary Care for Physician Assistants*. New York, McGraw-Hill, 1998, chap 4–8.]

4-9. The correct answer is E. Lithium is not bound by activated charcoal, which is given only to patients suspected of having coingested other substances. The other overdoses are correctly paired with their respective antidotes or treatments. [Newell KA: Poisoning and overdose, in Moser RL (ed): *Primary Care for Physician Assistants*. New York, McGraw-Hill, 1998, chap 4–8.]

4-10. The correct answer is B. Heroin belongs in the narcotic/analgesic group and is well known as a respiratory depressant. The other responses, miotic pupils, decreased gastrointestinal motility, bradycardia, and hypotension, are all changes seen with heroin overdose. [Newell KA: Poisoning and overdose, in Moser RL (ed): *Primary Care for Physician Assistants*. New York, McGraw-Hill, 1998, chap 4–8.]

4-11. The correct answer is E. Aspirin overdose is often treated initially with emesis to remove particulate matter (tablets) to minimize erosive gastritis. Infants less than 9 months old should not be given an emetic as they may not be able to protect their airways. Similarly, an unconscious person should not be given an emetic for the same reason. In hydrocarbon, strong acid, or alkali ingestion, emesis is contraindicated as it may increase tissue destruction of the esophagus and increase the risk of aspiration. [Newell KA: Poisoning and overdose, in Moser RL (ed): *Primary Care for Physician Assistants*. New York, McGraw-Hill, 1998, chap 4–8.]

4-12. The correct answer is E. Cocaine use has its major effect on the heart. It is often associated with cardiac ischemia, infarction, and arrest. The others listed are appropriately paired to their respective areas of injury. [Newell KA: Poisoning and overdose, in Moser RL (ed): *Primary Care for Physician Assistants*. New York, McGraw-Hill, 1998, chap 4–8.]

4-13. The correct answer is A. Shivering disappears at temperatures less than 32°C (89.6°F). This is considered to be mild to moderate hypothermia. Patients with severe hypothermia have lost the ability to self-generate heat. Hypotension, cardiac arrhythmias, altered mental status, and neurologic abnormalities are generally present in severe hypothermia. [Newell KA: Hypothermia and other cold injuries, in Moser RL (ed): *Primary Care for Physician Assistants*. New York, McGraw-Hill, 1998, chap 4–9.]

4-14. The correct answer is E. Mental impairment, extremes in age, intoxication, and endocrine abnormalities are all associated with increased risk for developing hypothermia. Similarly, some patients who may be especially vulnerable to hypothermia include the mobility impaired, those taking certain medications, the malnourished, and those suffering from sepsis. In the healthy population, hypothermia may be seen in those with inadequate clothing or exposed to severe weather conditions. [Newell KA: Hypothermia and other cold injuries, in Moser RL (ed): *Primary Care for Physician Assistants*. New York, McGraw-Hill, 1998, chap 4–9.]

4-15. The correct answer is D. Anhidrosis, or failure of perspiration, is a common finding in heat stroke. In cases of exertional heat stroke, however, sweating persists in up to 50 percent of the cases. [Smith JR: Heat stroke, in Moser RL (ed): *Primary Care for Physician Assistants*. New York, McGraw-Hill, 1998, chap 4–6.]

4-16. The correct answer is D. The diagnosis of heat stroke is, to a certain point, one of exclusion. Therefore, ruling out other causes of altered mental status coupled with high fever is crucial. CNS infection can present with symptoms similar to heat stroke. Overdosage of sympathomimetics such as cocaine and amphetamines may raise temperature and change mentation. Pheochromocytoma (adrenal tumor) will often produce catecholamine surges, which can raise temperature. Neuroleptic malignant syndrome is a relatively rare side effect of haloperidol therapy and can mimic heat stroke. Other potential differential diagnoses include cerebral falciparum malaria; overdosage of anticholinergics, salicylates, phenothiazines, butyrophenones, and thioxanthenes; withdrawal from amantadine, levodopa, and other dopaminergic medications; and thyroid storm. A meticulous medical history is critical in forming a complete and accurate differential diagnosis. [Smith JR: Heat stroke, in Moser RL (ed): *Primary Care for Physician Assistants*. New York, McGraw-Hill, 1998, chap 4–6.]

4-17. The correct answer is D. Fluid challenges are administered to comatose or semicomatose patients when the diagnosis is in doubt and risk of shock is increased. If, indeed, fluid deficit is wholly or partially responsible for the patient's condition, the challenge will aid in the diagnosis and help to assure an effective circulatory volume. [O'Connell CB: Disorders of fluid balance, in Moser RL (ed): *Primary Care for Physician Assistants*. New York, McGraw-Hill, 1998, chap 4–3.]

4-18. The correct answer is D. Packed red blood cells stay entirely in the vascular bed. Other fluids will distribute between the intracellular and extracellular fluid compartments. The divisions of the distribution will depend on the amount of solute. [Bennett JC, Plum F (eds): *Cecil Textbook of Medicine*, 20th ed. Philadelphia, Saunders, 1996, p 529.]

4-19. The correct answer is C. Of a liter of normal saline, about 300 mL will remain in the vascular bed, representing about a 6% increase in volume. [Bennett JC, Plum F (eds): *Cecil Textbook of Medicine*, 20th ed. Philadelphia, Saunders, 1996, p 529.]

4-20. The correct answer is B. Although tears are lost at 7% dehydration, when calculating fluid deficit needs it is recommended to round up to 10%. [O'Connell CB: Disorders of fluid balance, in Moser RL (ed): *Primary Care for Physician Assistants*. New York, McGraw-Hill, 1998, chap 4–3.]

4-21. The correct answer is D. Low body sodium can occur as a primary sodium loss or as a sodium and water loss. If more water than sodium is lost, a hypertonic state will occur. If more sodium than water is lost, a hypotonic state will occur. If the same proportion of water and sodium is lost, normal osmotic tension will remain. [Singer GG, Brenner BM: Fluid and electrolyte disturbances, in Fauci AS, Braunwald E, Isselbacher KJ, et al (eds): *Harrison's Principles of Internal Medicine*, 14th ed. New York, McGraw-Hill, 1998, pp 268–269.]

4-22. The correct answer is D. The kidneys respond to low-volume states by releasing ADH, which increases water reabsorption, and by activating the renin-angiotensin system to release aldosterone, which stimulates sodium retention in the tubules. Low-volume states are associated with tachycardia and a reduced effective circulatory volume. [Singer GG, Brenner BM: Fluid and electrolyte disturbances, in Fauci AS, Braunwald E, Isselbacher KJ, et al (eds): *Harrison's Principles of Internal Medicine*, 14th ed. New York, McGraw-Hill, 1998, pp 265–277.]

4-23.   The correct answer is D.   Hyponatremia is associated with increased muscle irritability, confusion, and possible seizure activity. Lethargy is common, especially in light of dehydration. Paralysis is more commonly seen in hypernatremic states. [Singer GG, Brenner BM: Fluid and electrolyte disturbances, in Fauci AS, Braunwald E, Isselbacher KJ, et al (eds): *Harrison's Principles of Internal Medicine*, 14th ed. New York, McGraw-Hill, 1998, p 269.]

4-24.   The correct answer is E.   Acidosis stimulates bicarbonate regeneration and reabsorption, stimulates respirations, and enhances ammonium production and excretion in order to enhance hydrogen secretion. [DuBose TD Jr: Acidosis and alkalosis, in Fauci AS, Braunwald E, Isselbacher KJ, et al (eds): *Harrison's Principles of Internal Medicine*, 14th ed. New York, McGraw-Hill, 1998, pp 277–286.]

4-25.   The correct answers are: anxiety: D; COPD: C; hyperventilation: D; milk-alkali syndrome: B; salicylate ingestion: A. [O'Connell CB: Acid-base disorders, in Moser RL (ed): *Primary Care for Physician Assistants*. New York, McGraw-Hill, 1998, chap 4–1.]

4-26.   The correct answer is C.   Acidosis drives hydrogen ions into the cells in exchange for potassium. Therefore, during the acute phase of diabetic ketoacidosis, serum potassium levels are commonly increased. The high potassium level stimulates potassium excretion by the kidneys as well, so that there may in fact be a low total body store of potassium regardless of the high serum level. [Bennett JC, Plum F (eds): *Cecil Textbook of Medicine*, 20th ed. Philadelphia, Saunders, 1996, p 542; Foster DW: Diabetes mellitus, in Fauci AS, Braunwald E, Isselbacher KJ, et al (eds): *Harrison's Principles of Internal Medicine*, 14th ed. New York, McGraw-Hill, 1998, p 2073.]

4-27.   The correct answer is A.   Increased anion gap represents an abundance of anions other than chloride and bicarbonate. The "unmeasured" anions that make up the anion gap include albumin, lactate, pyruvate, phosphate, and sulfate. [Bennett JC, Plum F (eds): *Cecil Textbook of Medicine*, 20th ed. Philadelphia, Saunders, 1996, p 546.]

4-28.   The correct answer is C.   Dog bites account for 80 to 90 percent of the over 3 million animal bites every year. Cat bites have an incidence of 400,000 bites per year. Human bites are the third most common, with 4 to 23 percent of bite wounds. Snake bites have an incidence of about 8000 bites per year. [Rice R: Animal bites, in Moser RL (ed): *Primary Care for Physician Assistants*. New York, McGraw-Hill, 1998, chap 4–4.]

4-29.   The correct answer is D.   Although all the listed organisms may be isolated from infected cat bites, *Pasteurella multocida* is the most common isolate. [Rice R: Animal bites, in Moser RL (ed): *Primary Care for Physician Assistants*. New York, McGraw-Hill, 1998, chap 4–4.]

4-30.   The correct answer is B.   Cat bites carry a high incidence of infection from *Pasteurella multocida*. Erythromycin and cephalexin have poor activity against *P. multocida*. Penicillin has good activity against *P. multocida* but has poor coverage of *Staphylococcus aureus*. Of those listed, only amoxicillin-clavulanate provides adequate antimicrobial activity against *P. multocida, S. aureus,* and other pathogens normally associated with cat bites. [Rice R: Animal bites, in Moser RL (ed): *Primary Care for Physician Assistants*. New York, McGraw-Hill, 1998, chap 4–4.]

SECTION 5
ENDOCRINOLOGY

5. ENDOCRINOLOGY

QUESTIONS

DIRECTIONS: Each question below contains suggested responses. Choose the **one best** response to each question.

5-1. Which of the following statements is TRUE regarding the pathogenesis of type II diabetes?

(A) Viruses have been implicated as a probable cause.
(B) There is autoimmune destruction of pancreatic islet cells.
(C) Hyperinsulinemia may be present.
(D) Genetic factors may be at work, as evidenced by increased incidence in certain ethnic groups, particularly European-Americans and Asian-Americans.
(E) Excessive insulin receptors may be present, leading to inadequate circulating insulin levels.

5-2. Who may be diagnosed as diabetic immediately?

(A) 12-year-old girl with glycosuria, no symptoms
(B) 46-year-old obese man with random blood sugar 100, weight loss, and fatigue
(C) 16-year-old boy with random blood sugar 140, no symptoms
(D) 58-year-old woman with random blood sugar 220, fatigue, thirst, polyuria, weight loss, blurry vision
(E) 50-year-old man with random blood sugar 150, no symptoms

5-3. As part of their dietary education, which of the following should a diabetic be told?

(A) Carbohydrates must be completely excluded from the diet.
(B) Protein-derived calories should comprise 50 percent of the diet.
(C) High-fat diets will cause ketoacidosis.
(D) High-fiber diets will slow carbohydrate absorption.
(E) Simple sugars are more beneficial than complex carbohydrates such as starches.

5-4. Which of the following statements is TRUE regarding insulin therapy?

(A) Insulin therapy is always required for type I diabetics.
(B) Insulin therapy is never indicated for type II diabetics.
(C) Some type I diabetics will benefit from the combination of insulin plus sulfonylurea therapy.
(D) Regular insulin has a duration of action of about 24 h.
(E) NPH insulin is derived from pork or beef and should not be used for new diabetics.

5-5. Which of the following is TRUE regarding sulfonylurea therapy?

(A) Chlorpropamide has a very short half-life thus must be taken frequently throughout the day.
(B) Side effects include inappropriate secretion of antidiuretic hormone.
(C) These drugs are preferred over insulin in patients with hepatic or renal impairment.
(D) These drugs are the agents of choice for gestational diabetics.
(E) Type I diabetics should be tried on these drugs before insulin is initiated.

5-6. Which one of the following is a TRUE statement regarding infections in diabetics?

(A) *Pseudomonas* species commonly infect the eye, causing pain and discharge.
(B) Cholecystitis due to monilia (*Candida*) is common.
(C) Mucormycosis of the external ear is a frequent cause of deafness.
(D) Common infections include endocarditis, meningitis, and viral pneumonia.
(E) Infections heal slowly in diabetics because of impaired leukocyte function and inadequate circulation.

5-7. Diabetic ketoacidosis (DKA) is MOST likely to be precipitated by which of the following?

(A) infection
(B) inadequate food intake
(C) excessive exercise
(D) excessive sulfonylurea intake
(E) surreptitious use of insulin

5-8. Who is MOST likely to develop DKA?

(A) 14-year-old girl
(B) 57-year-old woman taking chlorpropamide
(C) 42-year-old woman taking glyburide
(D) 56-year-old man who is diet controlled
(E) 32-year-old woman discovered to have an insulinoma

5-9. Which laboratory abnormality is MOST likely to be found in diabetic ketoacidosis?

(A) Serum glucose <50
(B) Arterial pH >7.5
(C) Decreased $PaCO_2$
(D) Normal serum ketones but elevated urine ketones
(E) Normal serum glucose but extreme urinary glycosuria

5-10. Which of the following signs or symptoms of hypoglycemia is due to beta-adrenergic stimulation?

(A) obtundation and coma
(B) seizures
(C) motor incoordination
(D) sweating
(E) headache

5-11. Which is MOST important in the treatment of hypoglycemia?

(A) adequate fluid replacement
(B) intravenous insulin infusion
(C) administration of glucose, preferably intravenously
(D) exercise, to mobilize fats
(E) administration of fat, because it is a more concentrated source of calories than sugars

5-12. Which one of the following does NOT feature obesity in its specific symptomatology?

(A) Cushing's syndrome
(B) hypothyroidism
(C) Prader-Willis syndrome
(D) insulinoma
(E) all of the above

5-13. Which of the following is a contraindication to use of anorexic drugs for weight loss?

(A) hypertension
(B) pregnancy
(C) agitated states
(D) use of MAO inhibitors
(E) all of the above

5-14. The most sensitive test for hypothyroidism is

(A) TSH
(B) T_4
(C) T_3
(D) T_3RU
(E) radioiodine uptake and scan

5-15. The most useful test to follow replacement therapy in a hypothyroid patient is

(A) T_3RU
(B) TSH
(C) T_4
(D) thyroglobulin
(E) T_3

5-16. The best replacement therapy for hypothyroidism is

(A) triiodothyronine
(B) desiccated thyroid
(C) a combination of T_4 and T_3
(D) iodine
(E) levothyroxine

5-17. The most common cause of hypothyroidism is

(A) thyroid surgery
(B) radioiodine ablation
(C) autoimmune thyroiditis
(D) discontinuation of prolonged levothyroxine therapy
(E) subacute thyroiditis

5-18. Which is characteristic of hypothyroidism?

(A) sweating
(B) increased appetite
(C) nervousness
(D) delayed relaxation of deep tendon reflexes
(E) low cholesterol

5-19. Hyperthyroidism associated with exophthalmos is MOST likely caused by

(A) toxic multinodular goiter
(B) subacute thyroiditis
(C) Hashimoto's thyroiditis
(D) exogenous thyroid hormone
(E) Graves' disease

5-20. Treatment of Graves' disease may include all the following EXCEPT

(A) methimazole
(B) radioactive iodine
(C) propranolol
(D) NSAID
(E) surgery

5-21. Which of the following laboratory abnormalities is NOT associated with Graves' hyperthyroidism?

(A) high TSH
(B) high T_4
(C) high radioiodine uptake
(D) high T_3
(E) diffuse pattern on thyroid scan

5-22. Which of the following may be useful in the treatment of hyperthyroidism associated with subacute thyroiditis?

(A) methimazole
(B) propylthiouracil
(C) propranolol
(D) radioiodine
(E) surgery

5-23. What advice should be given to a patient on propylthiouracil who develops fever and oral ulcers?

(A) increase the propylthiouracil dose
(B) discontinue propylthiouracil
(C) add levothyroxine
(D) add an NSAID
(E) give urgent radioiodine therapy

5-24. Addison's disease is characterized by

(A) low ACTH, low cortisol, normal aldosterone
(B) high ACTH, high cortisol, normal aldosterone
(C) high ACTH, normal cortisol, high aldosterone
(D) high ACTH, low cortisol, low aldosterone
(E) low ACTH, high cortisol, low aldosterone

5-25. The MOST common cause of secondary adrenal glucocorticoid deficiency is

(A) postpartum pituitary infarction
(B) high-dose ACTH administration
(C) tuberculosis
(D) Addison's disease
(E) prolonged high-dose glucocorticoid administration

5-26. Which is NOT a characteristic of Cushing's syndrome?

(A) hypertension
(B) hypoglycemia
(C) osteoporosis
(D) central obesity
(E) muscle wasting

5-27. Primary hyperaldosteronism is characterized by

(A) high renin, high aldosterone, low potassium
(B) low renin, low aldosterone, high potassium
(C) high renin, high aldosterone, high potassium
(D) low renin, low aldosterone, low potassium
(E) low renin, high aldosterone, low potassium

5-28. Secondary hyperaldosteronism with hypertension occurs with

(A) congestive heart failure
(B) renal artery stenosis
(C) nephrotic syndrome
(D) dehydration
(E) aldosterone-producing adenoma

5-29. Which is the MOST common cause of Cushing's syndrome?

(A) ACTH-producing pituitary tumor
(B) adrenal carcinoma
(C) adrenal adenoma
(D) ectopic ACTH-producing tumor
(E) none of the above

5-30. Hyperaldosteronism should be considered in patients with

(A) hypokalemia
(B) hyperkalemia
(C) hyponatremia
(D) hypernatremia
(E) acidosis

5-31. The secretion of parathyroid hormone is inhibited by

(A) lithium
(B) hypermagnesemia
(C) hypercalcemia
(D) hypovitaminosis D
(E) hypocalcemia

5-32. The most common cause of hypercalcemia is

(A) hypervitaminosis D
(B) secondary hyperparathyroidism
(C) malignancy
(D) parathyroid adenoma
(E) immobility

5-33. Increased parathyroid hormone is seen in

(A) malignancy
(B) vitamin D intoxication
(C) breast cancer
(D) fracture in Paget's disease
(E) primary hyperparathyroidism

5-34. A 45-year-old woman with an abnormal mammogram and a positive family history of breast cancer has hypercalcemia and an elevated serum parathyroid hormone level. The probable cause of hypercalcemia is

(A) breast cancer metastases
(B) primary hyperparathyroidism
(C) increased intestinal absorption of calcium
(D) inactivity because of bone pain
(E) increased parathyroid hormone–related protein

5-35. The pituitary hormone MOST commonly oversecreted by an adenoma is

(A) growth hormone
(B) prolactin
(C) ACTH
(D) TSH
(E) FSH

5-36. The MOST important hormone to replace in treating complete panhypopituitarism is

(A) cortisol
(B) thyroxine
(C) growth hormone
(D) estrogen or testosterone
(E) prolactin

5-37. Hypopituitarism may occur after which of the following?

(A) pregnancy
(B) pituitary surgery
(C) infarction of pituitary tumor
(D) trauma
(E) all of the above

5-38. Central diabetes insipidus is characterized by each of the following EXCEPT

(A) increased urine output
(B) hypernatremia
(C) low serum osmolality
(D) dilute urine
(E) decreased arginine vasopressin

5-39. Central diabetes insipidus is NOT caused by

(A) head trauma
(B) inherited defect
(C) hypothalamic tumors
(D) lithium
(E) pituitary surgery

5-40. The diagnosis of central diabetes insipidus is suggested by

(A) increased urinary osmolality
(B) hyponatremia
(C) decreased serum osmolality during water deprivation
(D) decreased urine concentration in response to arginine vasopressin
(E) persistently low urine osmolality during water deprivation

5-41. Treatment of central diabetes insipidus includes

(A) dialysis
(B) water restriction
(C) salt restriction
(D) desmopressin
(E) pituitary surgery

5-42. The syndrome of inappropriate antidiuretic hormone (ADH) is characterized by

(A) increased serum osmolality
(B) dilute urine
(C) hyponatremia
(D) renal insensitivity to arginine vasopressin
(E) edema

5-43. The treatment of the syndrome of inappropriate ADH includes

(A) nasal desmopressin
(B) rapid infusion of normal saline
(C) cautious infusion of 5% dextrose in water
(D) water deprivation
(E) rapid infusion of hypertonic saline if the serum sodium is less than 125 meq/L

5-44. Osteoporosis is characterized by

  (A) decreased bone mineralization
  (B) decreased bone mass
  (C) decreased bone resorption
  (D) increased serum calcium
  (E) decreased bone remodeling

5-45. Low peak bone mass is NOT associated with

  (A) menopause
  (B) calcium intake
  (C) activity
  (D) gender
  (E) ethnicity

5-46. Secondary osteoporosis is NOT seen in

  (A) thyrotoxicosis
  (B) Cushing's disease
  (C) calcium carbonate therapy for peptic ulcer disease
  (D) men treated with orchiectomy for prostate cancer
  (E) quadriplegia

5-47. The BEST test to demonstrate decreased bone density is

  (A) dual-photon densitometry
  (B) dual-energy x-ray absorptiometry
  (C) lateral x-ray of the spine
  (D) quantitative CT scan

5-48. Which is NOT indicated for treatment of a hypogonadal man with decreased bone density?

  (A) calcium
  (B) vitamin D
  (C) testosterone
  (D) regular light exercise
  (E) sodium fluoride

5-49. Paget's disease causes

  (A) diffuse demineralization of bone
  (B) pain
  (C) low serum calcium
  (D) low alkaline phosphatase
  (E) low cardiac output

5-50. The MOST dangerous complication of Paget's disease is

  (A) osteosarcoma
  (B) hypercalcemia
  (C) hypocalcemia
  (D) congestive heart failure
  (E) kidney stones

5. ENDOCRINOLOGY

ANSWERS

5-1. The correct answer is C. Hyperinsulinemia may be seen in type II diabetics. Still, there is a relative lack of insulin due to insulin resistance in obesity and decreased numbers of insulin receptors. [Herbert-Carter J: Diabetes mellitus, in Moser RL (ed): *Primary Care for Physician Assistants*. New York, McGraw-Hill, 1998, chap 5–1.]

5-2. The correct answer is D. This is the only patient that fits the diagnostic criteria:
1. Random blood glucose >200 with symptoms *or*
2. Fasting blood glucose >120 on more than one occasion *or*
3. Abnormal glucose tolerance test (GTT)

Remember that urine glucose tests, while they may be suggestive, are never adequate for diagnosis. [Herbert-Carter J: Diabetes mellitus, in Moser RL (ed): *Primary Care for Physician Assistants*. New York, McGraw-Hill, 1998, chap 5–1.]

5-3. The correct answer is D. The commonly prescribed diabetic diet provides 55 to 60 percent of calories from carbohydrates (preferably complex carbohydrates, i.e., starches and fruits), 10 to 20 percent from proteins, and 25 to 30 percent from fats. High fiber is recommended (25g/1000 kcal) to slow absorption of sugars. [Herbert-Carter J: Diabetes mellitus, in Moser RL (ed): *Primary Care for Physician Assistants*. New York, McGraw-Hill, 1998, chap 5–1.]

5-4. The correct answer is A. Insulin is an absolute requirement for type I diabetics and is also sometimes used for type II diabetics. Oral agents work by increasing pancreatic insulin secretion. Thus, in a pancreas without islet cells, they will be ineffective. Persons started on insulin several years ago may still be using pork or beef preparations. However, as a general rule, diabetics starting insulin for the first time should receive one of the human insulin preparations. Use of human insulin affords less risk of allergy, immune-based resistance, and local reactions such as lipoatrophy.

Most commonly used insulin preparations (whether animal derived or human via recombinant DNA technology) are "regular" (or "R"), which is short acting, and NPH (or "N"), which is considered intermediate acting. NPH is mixed with a protein and the NPH (or "N"), considered intermediate acting. NPH is mixed with a protein and the pH adjusted to provide longer-term coverage. Regular insulin has an onset of action within about 1/2 h when injected subcutaneously, peak action in 2 to 4 h, and a duration of about 6 to 8 h. NPH has onset in about 2 to 4 h, peak in 6 to 8 h, and duration about 18 to 24 h. [Herbert-Carter J: Diabetes mellitus, in Moser RL (ed): *Primary Care for Physician Assistants*. New York, McGraw-Hill, 1998, chap 5–1.]

5-5. The correct answer is B. Sulfonylureas may be divided into first- and second-generation agents. The most commonly used first-generation agent is chlorpropamide. The daily dose ranges from 100 to 500 mg given in the morning. It has an extremely long duration of action: 60 h. Adverse effects include an Antabuse-like effect and inappropriate secretion of antidiuretic hormone (SIADH). The long duration of action makes once-daily dosing convenient. However, when problems occur, e.g., hypoglycemia in a poorly nourished elderly patient, clearance of the drug is very slow, prolonging the problematic situation.

Second-generation sulfonylureas are glipizide (Glucotrol) and glyburide (DiaBeta, Micronase). These are used in dosages of 2.5 to 40 mg daily with duration of action of 12 to 24 h. Their mechanisms of action, contraindications, etc., are similar to the first generation's.

Oral hypoglycemics (sulfonylureas) are often used for type II diabetics when diet alone is insufficient, but are never used for type I diabetics. Oral agents work by increasing pancreatic insulin secretion. Sulfonylureas are contraindicated in gestational diabetes, in hepatic or renal insufficiency, and for patients with allergy to sulfa drugs. [Herbert-Carter J: Diabetes mellitus, in Moser RL (ed): *Primary Care for Physician Assistants*. New York, McGraw-Hill, 1998, chap 5–1.]

5-6. The correct answer is E. Diabetics are prone to the same acute infections as the general population, but are also susceptible to several unusual infections. Malignant *Pseudomonas* otitis externa may be very serious because it may spread through the mastoid area and infect the sinuses and brain. Rhinocerebral mucormycosis, seen in ketoacidosis, is a fungal infection that may also spread through the nose and sinuses to infect the brain. It begins with a severe headache and nasal discharge but may end in coma and death. Amphotericin B is the drug of choice, with surgical debridement also necessary. Other infections seen more frequently in diabetics include emphysematous cholecystitis, necrotizing fasciitis, chronic osteomyelitis, and *Candida* (monilia) skin infections. [Herbert-Carter J: Diabetes mellitus, in Moser RL (ed): *Primary Care for Physician Assistants*. New York, McGraw-Hill, 1998, chap 5–1.]

5-7. The correct answer is A. This is the only choice that is likely to precipitate DKA. All the other choices are causes of hypoglycemia. [Herbert-Carter J: Diabetic ketoacidosis, in Moser RL (ed): *Primary Care for Physician Assistants*. New York, McGraw-Hill, 1998, chap 5–7.]

5-8. The correct answer is A. Type I diabetics are more likely to develop DKA than type II diabetics. Only the 14-year-old child is likely to be a type I diabetic. [Herbert-Carter J: Diabetic ketoacidosis, in Moser RL (ed): *Primary Care for Physician Assistants*. New York, McGraw-Hill, 1998, chap 5–7.]

5-9. The correct answer is C. Serum ketones are invariably present. Hyperglycemia is also present. It is commonly extreme, but sometimes only moderate. Urine ketones may be negative. The common urine tests for ketones only check for acetoacetate, while the predominant one in DKA is beta hydroxybutyrate. Arterial blood gases will demonstrate acidosis (pH <7.4). There will be low $PaCO_2$ because of tachypnea (a compensatory mechanism due to the metabolic acidosis). Electrolytes will demonstrate an increased anion-gap acidosis. Electrolyte abnormalities are variable because the degree of dehydration and hyperglycemia will affect measured values for sodium, potassium, and phosphate. [Herbert-Carter J: Diabetic ketoacidosis, in Moser RL (ed): *Primary Care for Physician Assistants*. New York, McGraw-Hill, 1998, chap 5–7.]

5-10. The correct answer is D. The hypoglycemic patient may complain of sweating, palpitations, hunger, tremor, nervousness, and weakness. These all result from stimulation of the beta-adrenergic system (epinephrine). These signs may be blunted or absent in the patient taking beta blockers, such as propanolol (Inderal). Patients may have lightheadedness, diplopia, headache, motor incoordination, confusion, obtundation, seizures, and coma. These result from glucose starvation in the central nervous system. [Herbert-Carter J: Insulin shock (hypoglycemia), in Moser RL (ed): *Primary Care for Physician Assistants*. New York, McGraw-Hill, 1998, chap 5–8.]

5-11. The correct answer C. Intravenous glucose (dextrose) is the treatment for hypoglycemia. In early stages, an alert patient may notice tremulousness, hunger, sweating, and palpitations and be able to take oral glucose or simply food. Absorption is not guaranteed and onset of action may be delayed. Thus, intravenous glucose is always best, when available. The comatose patient will awaken quickly if hypoglycemia has not gone so long that permanent brain damage has occurred. Even with rapid awakening, the hypoglycemic patient must be carefully monitored. Remember the long half-life of the sulfonylureas. If these are the cause of the hypoglycemia, repeat attacks may occur after correction, and repeat therapy may be needed. [Herbert-Carter J: Insulin shock (hypoglycemia), in Moser RL (ed): *Primary Care for Physician Assistants*. New York, McGraw-Hill, 1998, chap 5–8.]

5-12. **The correct answer is E.** All answers are correct as being secondary causes of obesity. Cushing's with centripetal fat stores, along with insulinoma that causes obesity from increased energy intake secondary to recurrent hypoglycemia, are examples. Prader-Willis syndrome is a rare disorder thought to be hypothalamic in origin. [Paterson KB: Obesity, in Moser RL (ed): *Primary Care for Physician Assistants*. New York, McGraw-Hill, 1998, chap 5–12.]

5-13. **The correct answer is E.** The list of contraindications for using this class of obesity (anorexic) drugs is extensive. Patients should not be started on these medications without previous screening, which should include a complete physical and laboratory, and close management is essential. Other possible secondary causes of obesity should first be ruled out before medication is started. [Paterson KB: Obesity, in Moser RL (ed): *Primary Care for Physician Assistants*. New York, McGraw-Hill, 1998, chap 5–12.]

5-14. **The correct answer is A.** In all patients but those few cases of hypothyroidism caused by pituitary TSH deficiency, pituitary secretion of TSH is the most sensitive test of hypothyroidism, since it is essentially an internal bioassay of the patient's circulating free thyroid hormone level. T_4 with T_3RU is useful, but T_3 and radioiodine uptake and scan are not. [Evans TC: Hypothyroidism, in Moser RL (ed): *Primary Care for Physician Assistants*. New York, McGraw-Hill, 1998, chap 5–3.]

5-15. **The correct answer is B.** Once hypothyroidism has been diagnosed, TSH is the most useful, and in most cases the only, test to follow replacement therapy. In essence, the pituitary is serving as an internal biological assay of the amount of circulating free thyroid hormone. [Evans TC: Hypothyroidism, in Moser RL (ed): *Primary Care for Physician Assistants*. New York, McGraw-Hill, 1998, chap 5–3.]

5-16. **The correct answer is E.** Levothyroxine is well-standardized, reliable, and the only necessary replacement therapy for hypothyroidism. T_4 is converted as needed to T_3 in the body by normal processes. The long half-life of T_4, compared with T_3 (which is also present in desiccated thyroid), ensures smooth blood levels and no harmful consequences of an occasional missed dose. Iodine would only be effective in iodine-deficient areas of the world. [Evans TC: Hypothyroidism, in Moser RL (ed): *Primary Care for Physician Assistants*. New York, McGraw-Hill, 1998, chap 5–3.]

5-17. **The correct answer is C.** Autoimmune thyroiditis (Hashimoto's thyroiditis) is by far the most common cause of hypothyroidism. Thyroidectomy and radioiodine ablation cause permanent hypothyroidism and transient hypothyroidism occurs during the recovery phase of subacute thyroiditis. After discontinuation of thyroid replacement therapy, a normal thyroid will again resynthesize and secrete normal amounts of thyroid hormone in response to rising TSH levels. [Evans TC: Hypothyroidism, in Moser RL (ed): *Primary Care for Physician Assistants*. New York, McGraw-Hill, 1998, chap 5–3.]

5-18. **The correct answer is D.** Physical findings in hypothyroidism may include lethargy, dry puffy skin, hair loss, and characteristic delay of the relaxation phase of deep tendon reflexes. Sweating, increased appetite, and nervousness are characteristic of hyperthyroidism. Hypothyroidism is associated with increased cholesterol. [Evans TC: Hypothyroidism, in Moser RL (ed): *Primary Care for Physician Assistants*. New York, McGraw-Hill, 1998, chap 5–3.]

5-19. **The correct answer is E.** Each of these choices may cause thyrotoxicosis. Technically, exogenous thyroid hormone can cause thyrotoxicosis but not hyperthyroidism, since the excess thyroid hormone does not come from the thyroid gland. Only Graves' disease is associated with exophthalmos. [Evans TC: Hyperthyroidism, in Moser RL (ed): *Primary Care for Physician Assistants*. New York, McGraw-Hill, 1998, chap 5–4.]

5-20. **The correct answer is D.** The overactivity of the thyroid in Graves' disease can be inhibited with methimazole or propylthiouracil. Propranolol is useful to dampen the catecholaminergic symptoms of marked thyrotoxicosis. Either radioiodine or surgery can be used to ablate the thyroid. Anti-inflammatory drugs have no role in the treatment of Graves' disease. [Evans TC: Hyperthyroidism, in Moser RL (ed): *Primary Care for Physician Assistants*. New York, McGraw-Hill, 1998, chap 5–4.]

5-21. **The correct answer is A.** The high T_4 and T_3 of Graves' disease suppress pituitary TSH secretion. The overactivity of the gland is shown by the high radioiodine uptake and the generalized nature of the thyroid disease is shown by the diffuse pattern of increased uptake on the scan. [Evans TC: Hyperthyroidism, in Moser RL (ed): *Primary Care for Physician Assistants*. New York, McGraw-Hill, 1998, chap 5–4.]

5-22. **The correct answer is C.** The increased thyroid hormone seen in subacute thyroiditis is released from the thyroid during the time of acute inflammation. It is not produced by thyroid overactivity. Therefore, therapy directed at decreasing thyroid overactivity, such as antithyroid drugs and radioiodine, is ineffective in subacute thyroiditis. Propranolol is useful to decrease catecholamine-related symptoms such as tachycardia and tremor. Surgery is not necessary for subacute thyroiditis. [Evans TC: Hyperthyroidism, in Moser RL (ed): *Primary Care for Physician Assistants*. New York, McGraw-Hill, 1998, chap 5–4.]

5-23. **The correct answer is B.** The most serious side effect of propylthiouracil and methimazole is agranulocytosis, which usually resolves spontaneously when the drug is discontinued. Warning signs include oral ulcers, fever, and infections. [Evans TC: Hyperthyroidism, in Moser RL (ed): *Primary Care for Physician Assistants*. New York, McGraw-Hill, 1998, chap 5–4.]

5-24. **The correct answer is D.** Addison's disease is primary adrenal insufficiency caused by autoimmune inflammation of the adrenal cortex. As such, the cells that produce aldosterone as well as the cortisol-producing cells are destroyed. Therefore, both hormones are low. ACTH is elevated because of absence of cortisol feedback inhibition on the pituitary. [Evans TC: Adrenal disorders, in Moser RL (ed): *Primary Care for Physician Assistants*. New York, McGraw-Hill, 1998, chap 5–5.]

5-25. **The correct answer is E.** Secondary adrenal glucocorticoid deficiency results from insufficient adrenal stimulation by pituitary ACTH. By far the most common cause of pituitary ACTH deficiency is prolonged glucocorticoid administration. High-dose glucocorticoid administration for as little as a few weeks can result in prolonged pituitary ACTH suppression and, therefore, lack of adrenal cortisol production. [Evans TC: Adrenal disorders, in Moser RL (ed): *Primary Care for Physician Assistants*. New York, McGraw-Hill, 1998, chap 5–5.]

5-26. **The correct answer is B.** Excess cortisol opposes the action of insulin and causes hyperglycemia, and sometimes overt diabetes mellitus. Other characteristic features of cortisol excess include characteristic body habitus with central obesity and muscle wasting, hypertension, osteoporosis, thin skin, easy bruising, menstrual abnormalities, hirsutism, and others. [Evans TC: Adrenal disorders, in Moser RL (ed): *Primary Care for Physician Assistants*. New York, McGraw-Hill, 1998, chap 5–5.]

5-27. The correct answer is E. In primary hyperaldosteronism, aldosterone is inappropriately produced by the adrenal cortex without normal stimulation by renin. This results in the abnormal combination of high aldosterone and low renin. The primary effect of aldosterone is renal retention of sodium in exchange for potassium. Thus, unprovoked hypokalemia is suggestive of hyperaldosteronism. [Evans TC: Adrenal disorders, in Moser RL (ed): *Primary Care for Physician Assistants*. New York, McGraw-Hill, 1998, chap 5–5.]

5-28. The correct answer is B. Renal artery stenosis results in renal underperfusion and increased renin production, which in turn causes increased aldosterone via increased angiotensin II. Congestive heart failure, nephrotic syndrome, and dehydration are all also associated with secondary hyperaldosteronism via increased renal renin production, but they are not hypertensive states. An aldosterone-producing adenoma is primary hyperaldosteronism—renin is low. [Evans TC: Adrenal disorders, in Moser RL (ed): *Primary Care for Physician Assistants*. New York, McGraw-Hill, 1998, chap 5–5.]

5-29. The correct answer is E. The most common cause by far of excess glucocorticoid is iatrogenic. Glucocorticoids are very commonly administered for allergic and inflammatory conditions such as reactive airway disease, rheumatoid arthritis, systemic lupus erythematosus, and many others. Of the other choices, ACTH-producing pituitary tumor is most common. The others are unusual. [Evans TC: Adrenal disorders, in Moser RL (ed): *Primary Care for Physician Assistants*. New York, McGraw-Hill, 1998, chap 5–5.]

5-30. The correct answer is A. The action of aldosterone is to increase renal reabsorption of sodium in exchange for potassium and hydrogen ions. Consequently, hyperaldosteronism causes hypokalemia and alkalosis. Hypernatremia does not occur because water is retained along with sodium. [Evans TC: Adrenal disorders, in Moser RL (ed): *Primary Care for Physician Assistants*. New York, McGraw-Hill, 1998, chap 5–5.]

5-31. The correct answer is C. The secretory activity of the parathyroid glands is responsive to the serum calcium. When calcium increases above a threshold level, parathyroid hormone secretion is inhibited. Hypocalcemia and hypovitaminosis D, by decreasing calcium absorption from the intestine, are stimuli for parathyroid hormone secretion. Lithium increases the setpoint for calcium inhibition of parathyroid activity. Hypomagnesemia decreases parathyroid secretion. Hypermagnesemia has no effect. [Evans TC: Parathyroid disorders, in Moser RL (ed): *Primary Care for Physician Assistants*. New York, McGraw-Hill, 1998, chap 5–10.]

5-32. The correct answer is D. Primary hyperparathyroidism and malignancy account for 90 percent of cases of hypercalcemia. Of these, primary hyperparathyroidism is much more common, and most cases of primary hyperparathyroidism are caused by single parathyroid adenomas. A less common cause is parathyroid hyperplasia involving all four parathyroids. An uncommon cause is parathyroid carcinoma. [Evans TC: Parathyroid disorders, in Moser RL (ed): *Primary Care for Physician Assistants*. New York, McGraw-Hill, 1998, chap 5–10.]

5-33. The correct answer is E. Each of these choices is a cause of hypercalcemia. Primary hyperparathyroidism is distinguished from almost all other causes of hypercalcemia by the inappropriate elevation of parathyroid hormone in the setting of hypercalcemia. [Evans TC: Parathyroid disorders, in Moser RL (ed): *Primary Care for Physician Assistants*. New York, McGraw-Hill, 1998, chap 5–10.]

5-34. The correct answer is B. Though breast cancer can cause hypercalcemia, only hyperparathyroidism, of the choices here, is associated with an elevated serum parathyroid hormone level. This patient may have more than one cause of hypercalcemia. [Evans TC: Parathyroid disorders, in Moser RL (ed): *Primary Care for Physician Assistants*. New York, McGraw-Hill, 1998, chap 5–10.]

5-35. The correct answer is B. The most common pituitary hormone oversecreted by tumor is prolactin, followed by growth hormone and ACTH. Tumors overproducing TSH, LH, and FSH are quite unusual. [Evans TC: Anterior pituitary disorders, in Moser RL (ed): *Primary Care for Physician Assistants*. New York, McGraw-Hill, 1998, chap 5–6.]

5-36. The correct answer is A. Cortisol and thyroxine are both essential for life, but cortisol is more rapidly life threatening when severely deficient. When both are deficient, cortisol should be replaced first, because thyroxine increases cortisol metabolism and can therefore worsen cortisol deficiency. [Evans TC: Anterior pituitary disorders, in Moser RL (ed): *Primary Care for Physician Assistants*. New York, McGraw-Hill, 1998, chap 5–6.]

5-37. The correct answer is E. Any of these events can result in hypopituitarism. Hypopituitarism after pregnancy, Sheehan's syndrome, has become less common than in the past with improved techniques for monitoring and replacing maternal blood and fluid loss at delivery. [Evans TC: Anterior pituitary disorders, in Moser RL (ed): *Primary Care for Physician Assistants*. New York, McGraw-Hill, 1998, chap 5–6.]

5-38. The correct answer is C. The hallmark of diabetes insipidus is production of large-volume dilute urine despite increased serum osmolality. Central diabetes insipidus is characterized by decreased production of arginine vasopressin. Infrequently, diabetes insipidus is nephrogenic (renal insensitivity to arginine vasopressin). [Evans TC: Posterior pituitary disorders, in Moser RL (ed): *Primary Care for Physician Assistants*. New York, McGraw-Hill, 1998, chap 5–11.]

5-39. The correct answer is D. Central diabetes insipidus is characterized by decreased posterior pituitary production of arginine vasopressin, which can be inherited, idiopathic, or a result of trauma or surgery. Lithium causes renal insensivity to arginine vasopressin (nephrogenic diabetes insipidus). [Evans TC: Posterior pituitary disorders, in Moser RL (ed): *Primary Care for Physician Assistants*. New York, McGraw-Hill, 1998, chap 5–11.]

5-40. The correct answer is E. Central diabetes causes persistently low urinary osmolality, even during water deprivation, despite increased serum osmolality. The diagnosis of central diabetes is then secured by demonstrating increased urinary osmolality in response to administration of the arginine vasopressin analog, desmopressin. [Evans TC: Posterior pituitary disorders, in Moser RL (ed): *Primary Care for Physician Assistants*. New York, McGraw-Hill, 1998, chap 5–11.]

5-41. The correct answer is D. In central diabetes insipidus, the abnormality is deficient arginine vasopressin from the posterior pituitary; renal responsiveness is normal. Treatment is, therefore, administration of an analog of arginine vasopressin, desmopressin. Desmopressin is conveniently administered as a nasal spray once or twice daily. [Evans TC: Posterior pituitary disorders, in Moser RL (ed): *Primary Care for Physician Assistants*. New York, McGraw-Hill, 1998, chap 5–11.]

5-42. The correct answer is C. Hyponatremia in the absence of edema and circumstances of salt loss such as diuretic use with free-water volume replacement describes the syndrome of inappropriate ADH. Excess arginine vasopressin secretion has many causes. Renal sensitivity to the increased arginine vasopressin is normal. [Evans TC: Posterior pituitary disorders, in Moser RL (ed): *Primary Care for Physician Assistants*. New York, McGraw-Hill, 1998, chap 5–11.]

5-43. The correct answer is D. In addition to treating the underlying cause of the inappropriate ADH, the correction of hyponatremia is best accomplished by water restriction. Infrequently, hypertonic saline may be required if the sodium is very low and symptomatic. However, the risk of too-rapid sodium correction can be an often fatal complication called central pontine myelinolysis. [Evans TC: Posterior pituitary disorders, in Moser RL (ed): *Primary Care for Physician Assistants*. New York, McGraw-Hill, 1998, chap 5–11.]

5-44. **The correct answer is B.** Osteoporosis is characterized by decreased bone mass. That is, both the mineral component and protein matrix are decreased. Decreased bone mineralization is osteomalacia. Laboratory tests are typically normal in osteoporosis. Bone remodeling is often increased, including increased bone resorption and bone formation, but resorption is greater than formation. [Evans TC: Osteoporosis, in Moser RL (ed): *Primary Care for Physician Assistants*. New York, McGraw-Hill, 1998, chap 5–2.]

5-45. **The correct answer is A.** Peak bone mass is achieved between 30 and 40 years of age, before the average age of menopause. Calcium intake in childhood and adolescence, and activity are both positively associated with peak bone mass. Men have higher peak bone mass than women, and blacks have higher bone mass than other ethnic groups. [Evans TC: Osteoporosis, in Moser RL (ed): *Primary Care for Physician Assistants*. New York, McGraw-Hill, 1998, chap 5–2.]

5-46. **The correct answer is C.** Calcium carbonate is a mainstay of prevention or treatment of osteoporosis. Excess thyroid hormone or glucocorticoid causes secondary osteoporosis. Hypogonadism and prolonged inactivity are also associated with decreased bone mass. [Evans TC: Osteoporosis, in Moser RL (ed): *Primary Care for Physician Assistants*. New York, McGraw-Hill, 1998, chap 5–2.]

5-47. **The correct answer is B.** Dual-energy x-ray absorptiometry (DEXA) is the bone densitometry test with greatest precision and lowest radiation dose to the patient. [Evans TC: Osteoporosis, in Moser RL (ed): *Primary Care for Physician Assistants*. New York, McGraw-Hill, 1998, chap 5–2.]

5-48. **The correct answer is E.** Each of these choices would help to decrease bone loss. Testosterone and fluoride both stimulate bone formation. However, fluoride has not been shown to decrease the fracture rate and may actually increase fracture rate because of abnormal mineralization structure despite the fact that bone mass increases. [Evans TC: Osteoporosis, in Moser RL (ed): *Primary Care for Physician Assistants*. New York, McGraw-Hill, 1998, chap 5–2.]

5-49. **The correct answer is B.** Paget's is most typically characterized by bone pain. The demineralization is localized to a lytic area or entire bone, but does not cross into other bones, though they may be independently involved. Calcium may be increased with inactivity. Alkaline phosphatase is increased, sometimes to very high levels. Pagetic bone is quite vascular and can result in high output cardiac failure if enough bone is involved with the disease. [Evans TC: Paget's disease, in Moser RL (ed): *Primary Care for Physician Assistants*. New York, McGraw-Hill, 1998, chap 5–9.]

5-50. **The correct answer is A.** Osteosarcoma occurs in about 1 percent of patients with Paget's disease. This malignancy is usually untreatable in patients with Paget's. Hypercalcemia and kidney stones occur, especially in immobilized or bedridden Paget's patients. High-output congestive heart failure can occur if sufficient bone is involved because of the increased vascularity of pagetic bone. Hypocalcemia is not associated with Paget's disease. [Evans TC: Paget's disease, in Moser RL (ed): *Primary Care for Physician Assistants*. New York, McGraw-Hill, 1998, chap 5–9.]

SECTION 6
GASTROENTEROLOGY

6. GASTROENTEROLOGY

QUESTIONS

DIRECTIONS: Each question below contains suggested responses. Choose the **one best** response to each question.

6-1. Which of the following is a characteristic finding of malabsorption syndromes?

(A) constipation
(B) melanic stools
(C) abdominal distention
(D) crampy abdominal pain
(E) large, loose, foul-smelling stools

6-2. The Schilling test is BEST used to evaluate which of the following?

(A) B_{12} deficiency
(B) fat malabsorption
(C) vitamin D deficiency
(D) vitamin K deficiency
(E) protein malabsorption

6-3. A 55-year-old man is seen with a 15-lb weight loss, watery diarrhea, and mild abdominal pain in the emergency department. He has a 45 pack/year history of tobacco abuse and alcohol abuse. Examination reveals a thin, pale male with muscle wasting. A flat plate of the abdomen shows epigastric calcifications. Which of the following is the MOST likely diagnosis?

(A) acute pancreatitis
(B) gastric carcinoma
(C) cholecystolithiasis
(D) peptic ulcer disease
(E) pancreatic exocrine insufficiency

6-4. A 27-year-old serviceman presents 6 months after a 2-year tour in Panama. He is complaining of explosive watery diarrhea, weakness, and paraesthesias. On exam his skin is rough and dry with areas of purpura and early muscle wasting. Complete blood count (CBC) reveals a megaloblastic anemia. Which of the following is the recommended treatment of this patient's problem?

(A) Lomotil 2 mg every 4 h for 1 week
(B) penicillin G 600,000 units IM bid for 10 days
(C) tetracycline 250 mg qid for 1 to 2 months

(D) cholestyramine 2 gm bid for 1 month
(E) Donnazyme 1,000 units 2 tablets prior to meals

6-5. Which of the following diet recommendations is appropriate to a patient with a malabsorption syndrome?

(A) high fat
(B) low protein
(C) high carbohydrate
(D) medium-chain triglyceride
(E) very low-density lipoprotein

6-6. All of the following can cause a bile salt insufficiency (malabsorption) EXCEPT

(A) intestinal obstruction
(B) bacterial overgrowth
(C) ileal resection
(D) liver disease
(E) amyloidosis

6-7. A 47-year-old man is seen with abdominal pain and distention for the last week. He has had several bouts of vomiting and a persistent nausea. His wife is complaining of his fetid mouth odor. There has been no jaundice, fever, or diarrhea. Which of the following is the MOST likely diagnosis?

(A) acute gastroenteritis
(B) hepatitis
(C) cholecystitis
(D) duodenal reflux
(E) bowel obstruction

6-8. Which of the following chemotherapeutic medications is considered the WORST for causing nausea and vomiting?

(A) dacarbazine
(B) Mithracin
(C) cisplatin
(D) 5-fluorouracil
(E) methotrexate

6-9. Which of the following is NOT considered a vascular source of nausea and vomiting?

(A) headaches
(B) hypertension
(C) mesenteric angina
(D) congestive heart failure
(E) acute myocardial infarction

6-10. Which of the following is the presumed mechanism of nausea in the presence of narcotics like codeine or morphine?

(A) irritability at the chemoreceptor trigger zone (CTZ)
(B) dampening the mediation of cranial nerve X
(C) production of localized gastric irritation
(D) reduction of gastric motility
(E) neurologic toxicity

6-11. Which of the following is LEAST likely to trigger an acute pancreatitis?

(A) hypertriglyceridemia
(B) cholecystolithiasis
(C) abdominal surgery
(D) ACE inhibitors
(E) pneumonia

6-12. Which of the following pain medications should be avoided in the treatment of acute or chronic pancreatitis?

(A) morphine
(B) ibuprofen (Motrin)
(C) ketorolac (Toradol)
(D) meperidine (Demerol)
(E) acetaminophen with codeine

6-13. Which of the following can be a distinguishing factor on physical examination for acute pancreatitis versus an acute abdomen?

(A) a soft, exquisitely tender abdomen
(B) positive orthostatic vital signs
(C) evidence of dehydration
(D) abdominal distention
(E) a quiet abdomen

6-14. Which of the following has been implicated in the etiology of peptic ulcer disease (PUD)?

(A) *Streptococcus pneumoniae*
(B) *Staphylococcus aureus*
(C) *Haemophilus influenzae*
(D) *Moraxella catarrhalis*
(E) *Helicobacter pylori*

6-15. Peptic ulcer disease is known for the classic symptom of deep, gnawing epigastric pain. What is the most common mechanism associated with the "silent" ulcer?

(A) frequent eating
(B) loss of vagus stimulation
(C) *Helicobacter pylori* infection
(D) use of over-the-counter H_2 blockers

6-16. What is the most common etiology of peptic ulcer disease in the elderly?

(A) alcohol abuse
(B) tobacco abuse
(C) use of NSAIDs
(D) use of steroids
(E) *Helicobacter pylori*

6-17. A 53-year-old man is seen with deep epigastric pain for 1 week. He has been chewing TUMS nonstop with little relief for the last 2 weeks. Last night he experienced dizziness and three black stools. On physical exam he is pale with positive orthostatic vital signs. Hemoccult testing is positive for blood. Which of the following would provide the most definitive diagnosis?

(A) abdominal ultrasound
(B) esophagogastroduodenoscopy (EGD)
(C) abdominal computerized tomograms (CT scan)
(D) barium upper gastrointestinal examination (UGI)
(E) endoscopic retrograde cholangiopancreatography (ERCP)

6-18. Which of the following does NOT commonly cause the development of a stress ulcer?

(A) burns
(B) renal failure
(C) polycythemia
(D) intracranial trauma
(E) severe dehydration

6-19. Which of the following is an appropriate therapy for the eradication of *H. pylori* infections?

(A) nizatidine 300 mg bid with Mylanta qid for 6 weeks
(B) bismuth compound qid with metronidazole (Flagyl) 250 mg tid for 3 weeks
(C) ranitidine 150 mg bid with tetracycline 250 mg tid for 10 days
(D) amoxicillin 250 mg tid with metronidazole 250 mg tid for 21 days
(E) omeprazole 20 mg bid and clarithromycin 500 mg tid for 14 days

6-20. Zollinger-Ellison syndrome is a hypersecretion of hydrochloric acid caused by the presence of

(A) gastrinomas
(B) amyloidosis
(C) liver disease
(D) *Helicobacter pylori*
(E) bacterial overgrowth

6-21. Pilonidal disease is caused by which of the following?

(A) perianal abscess from midline crypts
(B) foreign-body reaction from obstructing hair and keratin
(C) hidradenitis suppurativa
(D) furuncle

6-22. The MOST common location of pilonidal abscess or sinus tract is

(A) posterior
(B) anterior
(C) midline
(D) none of the above

6-23. In acute pilonidal abscess, which of the following is the appropriate therapy?

(A) antibiotics and moist heat
(B) incision and drainage, followed by immediate excision of sinus tract
(C) incision and drainage, allow time for infection to subside, followed by elective excision of sinus tract
(D) analgesics and wait for it to spontaneously rupture

6-24. Predisposing factors for the development of proctitis include all of the following EXCEPT

(A) inflammatory bowel disease
(B) male homosexuality
(C) pelvic radiation
(D) diverticulosis

6-25. A 32-year-old male presents with a 1-week history of severe rectal pain radiating to his buttocks, tenesmus, and difficulty urinating. On physical exam, draining perianal ulcers and vesicles are noted. These findings are MOST consistent with

(A) *Chlamydia* proctitis
(B) inflammatory proctitis
(C) herpes simplex proctitis
(D) *Campylobacter* proctitis

6-26. A 46-year-old female presents to the ER complaining of bloody diarrhea for 2 days. She reports a similar episode occurring 3 months ago that resolved spontaneously. Since that time, she has noted chronic fatigue and weight loss equivalent to 5 lb. Physical examination reveals rectal tenderness on digital examination with gross blood mixed with mucus and brown stool noted on the examination glove. These findings are MOST consistent with

(A) adenocarcinoma of the colon
(B) ulcerative proctocolitis
(C) amebiasis
(D) chemical proctitis
(E) none of the above

6-27. Which of the following statements is TRUE regarding proctitis?

(A) Proctitis commonly affects all segments of the descending colon in a skipped pattern.
(B) STD proctitis is more common in patients who engage in receptive anal intercourse.
(C) Ischemic bowel should be suspected in pediatric cases of proctitis.
(D) all of the above
(E) none of the above

6-28. Which of the following studies would be diagnostic in establishing the etiology of proctitis in a 42-year-old male bisexual patient?

(A) viral cultures of vesicular rectal lesions
(B) Gram stains of rectal smears for gonorrhea
(C) both are correct
(D) neither is correct

6-29. The treatment of choice for *Chlamydia* proctitis is

(A) ciprofloxacin 500 mg PO bid × 10 days
(B) doxycycline 100 mg PO bid × 10 days
(C) ampicillin 500 mg PO bid × 14 days
(D) metronidazole (Flagyl) 750 mg PO bid × 10 days

6-30. Hemorrhoids are commonly found in all the following positions EXCEPT

(A) left lateral
(B) right posterolateral
(C) right anterolateral
(D) right lateral

6-31. Current treatment options for internal hemorrhoids include all the following EXCEPT

(A) rubber band ligation
(B) Endo-Lase
(C) dietary modification
(D) excision of thrombus

6-32. A 30-year-old male presents with abdominal pain and vomiting. You make the diagnosis of acute viral hepatitis. Your patient management plan would include all of the following EXCEPT

(A) low-fat, high-carbohydrate diet
(B) avoidance of strenuous activity
(C) acyclovir
(D) patient education regarding infectivity

6-33. The single most important test that serves as an indicator of the severity of acute viral hepatitis is

(A) ALT
(B) AST
(C) HBsAG
(D) prothrombin time
(E) alkaline phosphatase

6-34. A 22-year-old dental assistant comes to your office after experiencing a needle stick from a used needle. She has never been vaccinated against hepatitis B virus. Your management of this patient during this visit would be

(A) HBIG (hepatitis B immune globulin) plus the first dose of hepatitis B vaccine
(B) HBIG and ask the patient to return in 1 month for the first dose of the hepatitis B vaccine
(C) HBIG and tell the patient there is no need for the HBV vaccine
(D) the first dose of HBV vaccine

6-35. Which of the following is the first-line therapy for fulminant ulcerative colitis (UC)?

(A) cyclosporine
(B) sulfasalazine
(C) methotrexate
(D) metronidazole
(E) adrenal steroids

6-36. A 36-year-old woman is seen with vague complaints of malaise, 15-lb weight loss and a low-grade fever on and off for 2 weeks. She reports watery diarrhea for the last 2 months. On exam she is a thin, pale woman in no acute distress. The rectal exam reveals two fissures and a small rectal abscess. CBC reveals a mixed anemia and a mildly elevated WBC count. Which of the following can be used as a first-line therapy for this patient's condition?

(A) penicillamine
(B) methotrexate
(C) cyclosporine
(D) metronidazole
(E) total parenteral nutrition

6-37. Which of the following conditions is often misdiagnosed in elderly patients who actually have inflammatory bowel disease?

(A) constipation
(B) diverticulitis
(C) cholecystitis
(D) infectious colitis
(E) irritable bowel syndrome

6-38. Which of the following more frequently occurs with Crohn's disease but rarely with ulcerative colitis?

(A) gallstones
(B) renal stones
(C) digital clubbing
(D) erythema nodosum
(E) inflammatory arthritis

6-39. Which of the following is the MOST common cause of obstruction in the elderly?

(A) incarcerated hernia
(B) cholecystolithiasis
(C) bowel carcinoma
(D) intussusception
(E) adhesions

6-40. A 73-year-old man is diagnosed with a "closed loop" volvulus. Which of the following is a potential serious consequence of this condition?

(A) watery diarrhea
(B) abdominal distention
(C) increased borborygmi
(D) vomiting of fecal matter
(E) bowel necrosis with bleeding

6-41. Which of the following is a common presenting symptom with high intestinal obstruction?

(A) belching
(B) vomiting
(C) distention
(D) constipation
(E) watery diarrhea

6-42. A 56-year-old mechanic is seen with abdominal pain and vomiting, which has been progressive for 3 days. On exam he has dry oral mucosa, orthostatic vital signs, absent bowel sounds, no distention, and an empty rectal vault. Flat plate of the abdomen reveals bowel immobility. Which of the following is the MOST likely diagnosis?

(A) adynamic paralytic ileus
(B) Crohn's disease
(C) diverticulitis
(D) carcinoma
(E) volvulus

6-43. The MOST important aspect of treatment for a bowel obstruction is

(A) providing total parenteral nutrition
(B) placement of a nasogastric (NG) tube
(C) fluid and electrolyte replacement
(D) performing an abdominal surgery
(E) placement of a rectal tube

6-44. A 21-year-old college student is seen with her fourth episode of crampy abdominal pain and bloating. She complains of three loose stools over the last 36 h. Previous episodes have been associated with test taking. There is no fever, chills, melena, steatorrhea, weight loss, or anorexia. Which of the following is the MOST likely diagnosis based on history?

(A) Crohn's disease
(B) infectious colitis
(C) Whipple's disease
(D) acute gastroenteritis
(E) irritable bowel syndrome (IBS)

6-45. Which of the following is the MOST common physical finding in a patient with irritable bowel syndrome?

(A) hypoactive bowel sounds
(B) no specific physical findings
(C) positive orthostatic vital signs
(D) abdominal distention with ascites
(E) evidence of muscle wasting and weight loss

6-46. Which of the following is the PRIMARY therapeutic goal in the treatment of irritable bowel syndrome?

(A) normalize bowel habits
(B) improve stress reduction
(C) follow a low-residual diet
(D) decrease exercise regimen

6-47. A 50-year-old manic-depressive with a long-standing diagnosis of irritable bowel syndrome is seen for intermittent watery diarrhea followed by periods of constipation. Up until 2 months ago she had minimal difficulties with her IBS. She was recently institutionalized. Which of the following is the BEST next step?

(A) start a GI workup
(B) reassure the institution's staff
(C) increase her exercise regimen
(D) prescribe additional anxiolytics
(E) increase the bulking agent to 3 teaspoonfuls bid

6-48. A common presentation of fecal impaction in an older person is with

(A) localized abdominal pain
(B) diarrhea
(C) rectal bleeding
(D) back pain

6-49. Impaction of the proximal colon is MOST likely with which of the following conditions?

(A) Alzheimer's dementia
(B) multiple sclerosis
(C) stroke
(D) adenocarcinoma of the colon

6-50. Treatment of a fecal impaction includes

(A) mineral oil enema
(B) irritant laxatives
(C) hot water enema
(D) soap suds enema

6-51. Which of the following population groups is MOST likely to develop gallstones?

(A) Asian females
(B) African females
(C) Caucasian males
(D) Middle Eastern males
(E) North American Indian females

6-52. Which of the following antibiotics has been implicated in the transient development of cholelithiasis?

(A) ampicillin/sulbactam (Unasyn)
(B) cefoperazone (Cefobid)
(C) ceftriaxone (Rocephin)
(D) tetracyclines

6-53. A 44-year-old woman is seen with 4 h of a steady severe pain in the right upper quadrant with radiation to the right shoulder. She is complaining of nausea without vomiting but has no fever, chills, diarrhea, cough, or chest pain. Examination reveals only tenderness over the 9th rib midclavicular line. Which of the following is the MOST likely diagnosis?

(A) hepatitis
(B) pancreatitis
(C) cholelithiasis
(D) lactose intolerance
(E) peptic ulcer disease

6-54. Which of the following is responsible for the vast majority of acute gastroenteritis (AGE) in adults?

(A) magnesium-based medications
(B) short-lived bacterial infections
(C) short-lived rotaviruses
(D) *Clostridium difficile*
(E) hyperthyroidism

6-55. Which of the following have been implicated in outbreaks of viral gastroenteritis in the last few years?

(A) strawberries
(B) raw oysters
(C) undercooked pork
(D) undercooked beef
(E) undercooked chicken

6-56. A 21-year-old student comes in with nausea, vomiting (four episodes), and diarrhea over the last 8 h. The symptoms woke him about 2:00 AM and he has been on or in front of the toilet every half hour until 8:00 AM. He is seeing you at 11:00 AM in the student clinic. The diarrhea was watery without melena or hematochezia. On exam he is pale and fatigued. He has borderline orthostatic vital signs and mild generalized abdominal tenderness. Which of the following is the MOST appropriate next step?

(A) send the patient home with a full liquid diet
(B) order stool cultures and stool for ova and parasites
(C) administer IV fluids for rehydration
(D) order a CT scan of the abdomen
(E) order enzyme immunoassays

6-57. Which of the following is the single BEST prevention of acute gastroenteritis?

(A) better governmental inspection of foods
(B) better refrigeration of prepared foods
(C) use of prophylactic antibiotics
(D) sterilized serving utensils
(E) good handwashing

6-58. Which of the following is considered the mainstay of gastroesophageal reflux disease (GERD) therapy?

(A) surgical repair
(B) 6 months of H$_2$ blocker therapy
(C) elimination of precipitating factors
(D) regular use of magnesium-based antacids
(E) 2-month course of a proton pump inhibitor

6-59. Which of the following medications requires yearly evaluations of the esophagus when used for the treatment of GERD?

(A) ranitidine (Zantac)
(B) cimetidine (Tagamet)
(C) omeprazole (Prilosec)
(D) aluminum-based antacids
(E) metoclopramide (Reglan)

6-60. A 63-year-old woman is seen with indigestion over the last 6 weeks. She has noticed an increasing fatigue and anorexia. Past medical history includes the diagnosis of hypertension, GERD, and non-insulin-dependent diabetes mellitus. She is currently taking Minipress and Metformin for control of her disease processes. She recently started using OTC antacids to help with the indigestion. She has excellent weight control and exercises regularly. Which of the following is the MOST appropriate next step?

(A) prescribe ranitidine (Zantac) bid for 3 months
(B) have her elevate the head of the bed up to 8 in
(C) refer for an immediate esophagogastroduodenoscopy
(D) reassurance and continued use of the OTC medications
(E) order a barium swallow, CBC, stool guaiac cards, and chemistries

6-61. A family is seen in the office with sudden onset of profuse watery diarrhea. Both adults and two children have mild epigastric pain. There was a family reunion picnic yesterday and they are not sure how fresh the food was. They have had no fever, nausea, vomiting, chills, hematochezia, or melena. Which of the following is the MOST likely cause of their colitis?

(A) *Yersinia*
(B) *Campylobacter*
(C) cytomegalovirus
(D) *Clostridium perfringens*
(E) *Histoplasma capsulatum*

6-62. Which of the following statements is TRUE regarding colorectal polyps?

(A) Seventy to eighty percent of polyps occur in the rectosigmoid colon.
(B) Most polyps are greater than 2 cm in diameter
(C) Most patients with colorectal polyps are asymptomatic.
(D) Polyps usually occur in clusters of 5 to 10 lesions.
(E) A and C

6-63. Clinical findings commonly associated with colorectal polyps include

(A) palpable abdominal mass
(B) profuse rectal bleeding
(C) positive stool for occult blood
(D) melanotic stools
(E) none of the above

6-64. Which of the following helps differentiate constipation from an acute abdominal event like cholecystitis?

(A) no weight loss
(B) pain is localized
(C) presence of tenesmus
(D) crampy abdominal pain
(E) lack of systemic symptoms

6-65. A 26-year-old woman comes in with intermittent, crampy left flank pain for the last 24 h. The pain is annoying but is getting progressively worse. Each cramping pain lasts about 20 s and comes about every 5 min. She has been traveling and admits to a poor diet and hydration. She has no fever, chills, nausea, vomiting, or diaphoresis. She reports one firm, brown stool 2 days ago. Which of the following would be the MOST EXPEDIENT diagnostic test for this patient?

(A) flat and upright abdominal films
(B) esophagogastroduodenoscopy (EGD)
(C) CT of the abdomen
(D) pelvic ultrasound
(E) barium enema

6-66. Which of the following medications is BEST known to cause constipation when used on a regular basis?

(A) tricyclic antidepressants
(B) B_{12} supplements
(C) alpha agonists
(D) ACE inhibitors
(E) nitrates

6-67. An elderly couple is heading for the Caribbean for a 10-day honeymoon. They have no known drug allergies. He has a history of peptic ulcer disease. What is the recommended prophylaxis for traveler's diarrhea?

(A) no prophylaxis is recommended
(B) amoxicillin 250 mg bid
(C) Keflex 500 mg daily
(D) Bactrim DS daily
(E) Ceftin 250 mg bid

6-68. Which of the following MOST OFTEN presents with a diarrhea state as its first symptom?

(A) cancer
(B) hepatitis
(C) cholecystitis
(D) HIV syndrome
(E) Whipple's disease

6-69. A 64-year-old woman is seen with several episodes of short, sharp, gripping LLQ abdominal pain. The initial sharp pain lasts about 30 s and is followed by 1 to 2 h of dull achy pain. Patient has had no constipation, diarrhea, fever, chills, weight loss, melena, or hematochezia. Physical exam is negative, including rectal exam. Which of the following is the MOST likely diagnosis?

(A) renal colic
(B) ovarian cyst
(C) diverticulosis
(D) colon carcinoma
(E) irritable bowel syndrome

6-70. Which of the following is considered the BEST exam to define diverticulosis?

(A) ultrasound
(B) sigmoidoscopy
(C) computer tomography
(D) barium enema with contrast
(E) magnetic resonance imaging

6-71. A 31-year-old woman is seen with a persistent chest fullness and pain for the last 5 weeks. She has noted a nocturnal cough and the inability to vomit. Physical examination is within normal limits except for a 10-lb weight loss. Which of the following is the MOST likely diagnosis?

(A) achalasia
(B) pyloric stenosis
(C) esophageal atresia
(D) peptic ulcer disease
(E) Zenker's diverticulum

6-72. A 42-year-old female presents with point tenderness just midway and inferior to the right inguinal ligament. You suspect

(A) direct inguinal hernia
(B) indirect inguinal hernia
(C) femoral hernia
(D) umbilical hernia
(E) ventral hernia

6-73. A common cause of appendicitis is

(A) fecal stasis and fecalith
(B) lymphoid follicular tissue
(C) tumors
(D) all of the above

6-74. All the following special exams can be performed to aid in the diagnosis of appendicitis EXCEPT

(A) Rovsing's sign
(B) psoas sign
(C) Kehr's sign
(D) obturator sign

6-75. Which of the following is the MOST common form of amebiasis in the United States?

(A) *Isospora belli*
(B) *Escherichia coli*
(C) *Cryptosporidium*
(D) *Entamoeba hartmanni*
(E) *Entamoeba histolytica*

6. GASTROENTEROLOGY

ANSWERS

6-1. The correct answer is E. The malabsorption of fat creates large, fluffy, frequent stools that often float and are malodorous. This may occur with acute gastroenteritis for short periods of time but is more commonly associated with chronic conditions like celiac sprue and Whipple's disease. [Heinly AP: Malabsorption, in Moser RL (ed): *Primary Care for Physician Assistants*. New York, McGraw-Hill, 1998, chap 6–18.]

6-2. The correct answer is A. A two-part test, the Schilling test is the best to evaluate B_{12}. A measured dose of radioactive B_{12} and an injection of nonlabeled B_{12} is delivered to the patient. If there is less than 8 percent of the measured radioactive B_{12} in urinary secretions, the malabsorption is confirmed. The next step is to administer intrinsic factor. Intrinsic factor is essential for the absorption of B_{12}. If the malabsorption corrects itself, it is the lack of intrinsic factor, not poor absorption, causing the deficiency. [Heinly AP: Malabsorption, in Moser RL (ed): *Primary Care for Physician Assistants*. New York, McGraw-Hill, 1998, chap 6–18.]

6-3. The correct answer is E. Often the result of chronic pancreatitis or repeated acute pancreatitis episodes, pancreatic exocrine insufficiency is the loss of pancreatic function (>90 percent). The loss creates malabsorption of fats, proteins, and carbohydrate creating diarrhea, weight loss, muscle wasting, and eventually ascites. The presence of epigastric calcification in the epigastrium is pathognomonic. [Heinly AP: Pancreatic disease, in Moser RL (ed): *Primary Care for Physician Assistants*. New York, McGraw-Hill, 1998, chap 6–20.]

6-4. The correct answer is C. This patient presents with tropical sprue. Common to the tropics, this disease may manifest years after leaving the area. Severe malnutrition and dehydration is common due to profuse diarrhea and electrolyte loss. Tetracycline dosing may extend out to 6 months and supportive care includes folic acid and Vitamin B_{12} replacement. [Heinly AP: Malabsorption, in Moser RL (ed): *Primary Care for Physician Assistants*. New York, McGraw-Hill, 1998, chap 6–18.]

6-5. The correct answer is D. The recommended diet is a high-protein, low-fat diet with emphasis on medium-chain triglycerides. The medium chains, from coconut oil, are easier to digest and absorb. [Heinly AP: Malabsorption, in Moser RL (ed): *Primary Care for Physician Assistants*. New York, McGraw-Hill, 1998, chap 6–18.]

6-6. The correct answer is E. Amyloid deposits in the intestinal mucosa cause a mucosal defect leading to malabsorption. Bile acid insufficiency is caused by liver disease (decreased production), bacterial overgrowth (excess use), ileal disease or resection (no reabsorption), and intestinal obstruction (poor reabsorption). Any disease that limits the bowel's access to bile acids can cause bile acid insufficiency. [Heinly AP: Malabsorption, in Moser RL (ed): *Primary Care for Physician Assistants*. New York, McGraw-Hill, 1998, chap 6–18.]

6-7. The correct answer is E. Bowel obstruction is a common cause of nausea and vomiting. The fetid breath is from bacterial overgrowth of the trapped intestinal secretions and waste. All the other choices are good differentials for this case. The distinction comes from the lack of systemic symptoms or findings. [Heinly AP: Intestinal obstruction, in Moser RL (ed): *Primary Care for Physician Assistants*. New York, McGraw-Hill, 1998, chap 6–16.]

6-8.   The correct answer is C.   Most chemotherapy induces some level of nausea because it causes a degree of gastric retention and renal and neurologic toxicity. Cisplatin is considered the worst for causing nausea; thus prophylactic antiemetic medications are usually given in conjunction with its use. [Heinly AP: Nausea and vomiting, in Moser RL (ed): *Primary Care for Physician Assistants*. New York, McGraw-Hill, 1998, chap 6–19.]

6-9.   The correct answer is B.   Acute myocardial infarction classically causes nausea. Hypotension or congestive heart failure can cause a low-grade but persistent nausea. Mesenteric angina and the other choices cause nausea by diversion or diminishment of blood supply to the GI tract. Headaches are also classic for nausea production due to the vascular involvement in the midbrain area. [Heinly AP: Nausea and vomiting, in Moser RL (ed): *Primary Care for Physician Assistants*. New York, McGraw-Hill, 1998, chap 6–19.]

6-10.   The correct answer is D.   Narcotics are notorious for producing nausea, especially in high doses. The presumed mechanism is the reduction of gastric motility. The slowed stomach retains contents that produce a full and nauseated sensation. The addition of a prokinetic like metoclopramide will counteract this effect so the patient can achieve pain control without nausea. The clinician should keep this common side effect and its remedy in mind. [Heinly AP: Nausea and vomiting, in Moser RL (ed): *Primary Care for Physician Assistants*. New York, McGraw-Hill, 1998, chap 6–19.]

6-11.   The correct answer is E.   Pneumonia may cause an elevation of amylase but is not a significant trigger of acute pancreatitis. By far the most common trigger is alcohol abuse. Some medications, such as ACE inhibitors and NSAIDs, have been implicated as triggers. Pregnancy, gallstones, and any obstruction of the ampulla of Vater can trigger acute pancreatitis by the sheer mechanics of blocking the egress of the pancreatic enzymes. [Heinly AP: Pancreatic disease, in Moser RL (ed): *Primary Care for Physician Assistants*. New York, McGraw-Hill, 1998, chap 6–20.]

6-12.   The correct answer is A.   Morphine is generally avoided because it is thought to cause spasm at the sphincter of Oddi (ampulla of Vater). The ductal spasm may increase obstruction of pancreatic juices and increase pain. [Heinly AP: Pancreatic disease, in Moser RL (ed): *Primary Care for Physician Assistants*. New York, McGraw-Hill, 1998, chap 6–20.]

6-13.   The correct answer is A.   Early acute pancreatitis is extremely painful with a soft abdomen. Severe pain with other acute abdomen conditions (appendicitis, diverticulitis, etc.) usually does not occur until there is significant guarding or a rigid abdomen. The mechanism appears to be extreme pain from autodigestion of pancreatic tissue before peritoneal signs can develop. The remainder of the signs may be common to any acute abdomen including pancreatitis. [Heinly AP: Pancreatic disease, in Moser RL (ed): *Primary Care for Physician Assistants*. New York, McGraw-Hill, 1998, chap 6–20.]

6-14.   The correct answer is E.   *H. pylori* is an S-shaped bacterium that infects the mucosal layer of the gastrium and duodenum. It is thought to cause up to 90 percent of all peptic ulcer disease. It produces urease, which in turn causes damage to the protective barriers of the mucosal layer. Effective eradication appears to cure PUD in the vast majority of patients. [Heinly AP: Peptic ulcer disease, in Moser RL (ed): *Primary Care for Physician Assistants*. New York, McGraw-Hill, 1998, chap 6–21.]

6-15.   The correct answer is D.   In the past, the most common reason for the "silent" ulcer with or without bleeding was frequent food intake. The food acts as a constant buffer against the acid, masking the pain. Today, the most common and concerning is the use of over-the-counter H$_2$ blockers. In low doses the pain may be avoided but the disease may progress. Ulcers take higher doses over a long period of time to heal completely. [Heinly AP: Peptic ulcer disease, in Moser RL (ed): *Primary Care for Physician Assistants.* New York, McGraw-Hill, 1998, chap 6–21.]

6-16. The correct answer is C. While up to 70 percent of the elderly may have an *H. pylori* infection, it is the use of nonsteroidal anti-inflammatory medications that causes the majority of peptic ulcers. The elderly are often treated with NSAIDs for aches and pain from arthritis, tendinitis, and the like. The antiprostaglandin effect is great for joints but is disruptive to the protective mechanisms of the intestinal mucosa. Additionally, the elderly are more prone to the silent ulcer because of a weakened immune system. [Heinly AP: Peptic ulcer disease, in Moser RL (ed): *Primary Care for Physician Assistants.* New York, McGraw-Hill, 1998, chap 6–21.]

6-17. The correct answer is B. An endoscopic exam allows for immediate investigation of bleeding sites and potential treatment with cautery. The direct visualization allows for biopsy and cultures. This patient is over 50 and symptomatic with pain, bleeding, and orthosis. These symptoms are sufficient for a rapid evaluation versus the time it would take for a UGI. A UGI may also produce false negatives or positives. While a CT scan or ultrasound might yield some information, it would not be definitive for ulcer disease. [Heinly AP: Peptic ulcer disease, in Moser RL (ed): *Primary Care for Physician Assistants.* New York, McGraw-Hill, 1998, chap 6–21.]

6-18. The correct answer is C. Polycythemia is an example of those diseases that may cause peptic ulcer disease because of a chronic change in blood supply or feedback mechanisms. Other diseases include cystic fibrosis, COPD, cirrhosis, and type 1 MEN. *Stress ulcers* occur due to a rapid shunting of the gastric blood supply to an area of injury. This shunting retards gastric mechanisms and feedback loops, causing injury and ulcers. [Heinly AP: Peptic ulcer disease, in Moser RL (ed): *Primary Care for Physician Assistants.* New York, McGraw-Hill, 1998, chap 6–21.]

6-19. The correct answer is E. Eradication of *H. pylori* is reliant on a medication combination being used consistently for 14 days. Another combination is bismuth compound 2 tablets qid, Flagyl 250 mg tid, with tetracycline or amoxicillin 500 mg tid for 14 days. The first combination has about an 80 percent cure rate and the second, which is harder to do, has about a 90 percent cure rate. The key is combination and compliance. [Heinly AP: Peptic ulcer disease, in Moser RL (ed): *Primary Care for Physician Assistants.* New York, McGraw-Hill, 1998, chap 6–21.]

6-20. The correct answer is A. Gastrinomas are most often reported in the pancreas, a non-beta cell tumor. They may also be found in the duodenum, spleen, and stomach. The gastrinomas produce a hypersecretion state in the gastrium leading to severe and recurrent gastric and duodenal ulceration. Zollinger-Ellison syndrome may be a component of multiple endocrine neoplasia type 1 (MEN 1) in up to 60 percent of cases. MEN type 1 is commonly associated with hyperparathyroidism. [Heinly AP: Peptic ulcer disease, in Moser RL (ed): *Primary Care for Physician Assistants.* New York, McGraw-Hill, 1998, chap 6–21.]

6-21. The correct answer is B. Perianal abscess from midline crypt describes an anal fistula. Hidradenitis suppurativa is an infection of the sweat glands. A furuncle is a boil. [Jan PCH: Pilonidal disease, in Moser RL (ed): *Primary Care for Physician Assistants.* New York, McGraw-Hill, 1998, chap 6–22.]

6-22. The correct answer is C. Pilonidal sinuses have a tendency toward the midline, where multiple cysts or sinus tracts can be found in the natal cleft. You see the characteristic tunnel with tufts of hair at some of the openings. [Jan PCH: Pilonidal disease, in Moser RL (ed): *Primary Care for Physician Assistants.* New York, McGraw-Hill, 1998, chap 6–22.]

6-23. The correct answer is C. Incision and drainage alone will not provide definitive treatment. Excision before infection has resolved may result in poor wound healing. [Jan PCH: Pilonidal disease, in Moser RL (ed): *Primary Care for Physician Assistants*. New York, McGraw-Hill, 1998, chap 6–22.]

6-24. The correct answer is D. Inflammatory bowel disease (ulcerative colitis) can involve the rectal mucosa exclusively. Male homosexuals practicing unprotected receptive anal intercourse are at increased risk for STD proctitis. A significant complication of radiation therapy to the pelvis is a severe proctitis resulting in fistulas and strictures. Symptoms may occur months to years after treatment. [Mayfield MS: Proctitis, in Moser RL (ed): *Primary Care for Physician Assistants*. New York, McGraw-Hill, 1998, chap 6–23.]

6-25. The correct answer is C. Both inflammatory proctitis due to ulcerative colitis and herpes simplex proctitis can cause rectal mucosal ulceration. However, only herpes simplex will present with perianal vesicular or ulcerated lesions and can involve the sacral nerve roots with paresthesias of the buttocks and thighs as well as bladder dysfunction. *Campylobacter* and *Chlamydia* infections do not cause perianal lesions. [Mayfield MS: Proctitis, in Moser RL (ed): *Primary Care for Physician Assistants*. New York, McGraw-Hill, 1998, chap 6–23.]

6-26. The correct answer is B. The majority of cases of amebiasis involve a noninvasive colitis. Patients are usually asymptomatic or develop symptoms of mild diarrhea and abdominal pain. Invasive infection with severe colitis and bloody diarrhea is rare. Adenocarcinoma of the colon may present with diarrhea, stool streaked with blood, or melena. Marked bleeding or bloody diarrhea is unusual. Chemicals in rectal suppositories or enemas can produce an irritative proctitis with mild to moderate inflammation of the rectum. Diarrhea and rectal bleeding usually do not occur. Recurrent bloody diarrhea, fatigue and weight loss are classic findings associated with ulcerative colitis. [Heinly AP: Colitis, in Moser RL (ed): *Primary Care for Physician Assistants*. New York, McGraw-Hill, 1998, chap 6–4.]

6-27. The correct answer is B. Proctitis is generally a disease localized to the rectal vault. Ischemic bowel is a complication seen more often in the geriatric population. Engaging in receptive anal intercourse is a high risk factor for STD proctitis. [Mayfield MS: Proctitis, in Moser RL (ed): *Primary Care for Physician Assistants*. New York, McGraw-Hill, 1998, chap 6–23.]

6-28. The correct answer is A. Patients who may engage in anal receptive intercourse should be worked up for an STD proctitis. Vesicular lesions noted are often due to herpes proctitis, which can be detected by Tzanck smear or viral cultures. Rectal cultures have a much higher yield than Gram stains for diagnosing gonorrhea. [Mayfield MS: Proctitis, in Moser RL (ed): *Primary Care for Physician Assistants*. New York, McGraw-Hill, 1998, chap 6–23.]

6-29. The correct answer is B. The preferred treatment for *Chlamydia* proctitis is doxycycline 100 mg PO bid × 10 days. Tetracycline may also be used. Ciprofloxacin is the recommended treatment for shigellosis/*Campylobacter* proctitis and is an alternative drug for gonorrhea proctitis. Metronidazole may be used to treat amebiasis. Ampicillin is not an effective agent for treating proctitis. [Mayfield MS: Proctitis, in Moser RL (ed): *Primary Care for Physician Assistants*. New York, McGraw-Hill, 1998, chap 6–23.]

6-30. The correct answer is D. Left lateral, right posterolateral, and right anterolateral positions are common locations for both internal and external hemorrhoids. Smaller hemorrhoids may appear at the right lateral position but it is not a common site for hemorrhoids. [Jan PCH: Hemorrhoids, in Moser RL (ed): *Primary Care for Physician Assistants*. New York, McGraw-Hill, 1998, chap 6–13.]

6-31. **The correct answer is D.** Internal hemorrhoids generally do not thrombose unless they prolapse beyond the anal verge and become incarcerated. External hemorrhoids typically thrombose and require excision for relief of pain. [Jan PCH: Hemorrhoids, in Moser RL (ed): *Primary Care for Physician Assistants*. New York, McGraw-Hill, 1998, chap 6–13.]

6-32. **The correct answer is C.** Acyclovir does not have antiviral activity against the hepatitis-causing viruses. A low-fat, high-carbohydrate diet is recommended for the patient with hepatitis and nausea and vomiting. Confinement in bed is not necessary, but rest is recommended. Hepatitis is a contagious disease and infectivity and means of transmission should be discussed. [Deasy J: Hepatitis, in Moser RL (ed): *Primary Care for Physician Assistants*. New York, McGraw-Hill, 1998, chap 6–14.]

6-33. **The correct answer is D.** The prothrombin test gives an indication of the degree of hepatic injury. The other tests listed do not. A prolonged prothrombin time can be an ominous sign. [Deasy J: Hepatitis, in Moser RL (ed): *Primary Care for Physician Assistants*. New York, McGraw-Hill, 1998, chap 6–14.]

6-34. **The correct answer is A.** HBIG provides protection via passive immunization until active immunization occurs from the hepatitis B vaccine. [Deasy J: Hepatitis, in Moser RL (ed): *Primary Care for Physician Assistants*. New York, McGraw-Hill, 1998, chap 6–14.]

6-35. **The correct answer is E.** With fulminant ulcerative colitis the goal is to decrease inflammation as soon as possible. Oral prednisolone may be used or IV prednisolone can be used if poor absorption is a problem. Sulfasalazine is used to control mild to moderate disease and should NOT be used for severe UC. Cyclosporine may be used for refractory UC, but it is not a first-line therapy. [Heinly AP: Inflammatory bowel disease, in Moser RL (ed): *Primary Care for Physician Assistants*. New York, McGraw-Hill, 1998, chap 6–15.]

6-36. **The correct answer is D.** Crohn's disease may be treated with metronidazole as a first-line therapy. It has been shown to be at least as effective as sulfasalazine. The sulfasalazine may be beneficial for colon disease but it has not been shown to be helpful with small intestinal disease. Steroids, cyclosporin, and methotrexate may be useful in severe disease. [Heinly AP: Inflammatory bowel disease, in Moser RL (ed): *Primary Care for Physician Assistants*. New York, McGraw-Hill, 1998, chap 6–15.]

6-37. **The correct answer is B.** Crohn's, in particular, has another peak incidence in the elderly, ages 60 to 80. In the elderly, diverticulitis may present with left lower quadrant pain, mass effect, and constipation. Irritable bowel syndrome may present the same but more commonly there is diarrhea. An index of suspicion is needed since the treatment of the two diseases is quite different. [Heinly AP: Inflammatory bowel disease, in Moser RL (ed): *Primary Care for Physician Assistants*. New York, McGraw-Hill, 1998, chap 6–15.]

6-38. **The correct answer is A.** Gallstone formation may be more common to Crohn's disease because of the frequent involvement of the distal ileum. The distal ileum is responsible for bile acid reabsorption—a critical element to bile juice equilibrium. A change in bile acid concentration can promote cholelithiasis. Ulcerative colitis very rarely involves the small intestine. The other choices are systemic manifestations that may occur with either disease. [Heinly AP: Inflammatory bowel disease, in Moser RL (ed): *Primary Care for Physician Assistants*. New York, McGraw-Hill, 1998, chap 6–15.]

6-39. **The correct answer is C.** The elderly are much more likely to develop obstruction from colon carcinoma, volvulus, and diverticulosis. The young person is more likely to have intussusception and incarcerated hernia. The most common small bowel obstruction is secondary to adhesion. [Heinly AP: Intestinal obstruction, in Moser RL (ed): *Primary Care for Physician Assistants*. New York, McGraw-Hill, 1998, chap 6–16.]

6-40. **The correct answer is E.** Bowel necrosis is much more common with twisting obstructions. As the obstruction persists there is intestinal wall edema, vasodilatation, increasing leakage, and fluid buildup. The progressive pressure and bacterial endotoxins cause bowel wall injury, necrosis, bleeding, and potential perforation. In the elderly this can result in death if not treated promptly. [Heinly AP: Intestinal obstruction, in Moser RL (ed): *Primary Care for Physician Assistants.* New York, McGraw-Hill, 1998, chap 6–16.]

6-41. **The correct answer is B.** Pain is the most common presenting symptom with small-intestinal obstruction, and vomiting a close second. Distention is more common in colonic obstruction, as is borborygmi. The fecal taste of vomitus is common to both due to bacterial overgrowth. [Heinly AP: Intestinal obstruction, in Moser RL (ed): *Primary Care for Physician Assistants.* New York, McGraw-Hill, 1998, chap 6–16.]

6-42. **The correct answer is A.** The key in this history is absent bowel sounds and lack of distention. The plain film will reveal no evidence of peristalsis and no dilated bowel loops or bird's beak finding common to small-intestinal mechanical obstructions. Crohn's disease may present with blurred haustral markings. [Heinly AP: Intestinal obstruction, in Moser RL (ed): *Primary Care for Physician Assistants.* New York, McGraw-Hill, 1998, chap 6–16.]

6-43. **The correct answer is C.** While you may execute on the other choices for any partic-ular patient, the essential is fluid support and correction of electrolyte imbalances. Dehy-dration and electrolyte disorders can lead to cardiac or brain events that can kill the patient before you can place an NG tube. Stick to the ABC's of resuscitation. [Heinly AP: Intestinal obstruction, in Moser RL (ed): *Primary Care for Physician Assistants.* New York, McGraw-Hill, 1998, chap 6–16.]

6-44. **The correct answer is E.** While IBS is a diagnosis of exclusion and cannot be made based on history alone, this is a classic presentation. The other choices are part of the dif-ferential diagnosis for IBS. The absence of systemic symptoms and weight loss is a vital clue. Also, the stress element may help differentiate, though not all IBS episodes are asso-ciated with stress. [Heinly AP: Irritable bowel syndrome, in Moser RL (ed): *Primary Care for Physician Assistants.* New York, McGraw-Hill, 1998, chap 6–17.]

6-45. **The correct answer is B.** Physical exam findings in a patient with irritable bowel syn-drome are usually absolutely *normal*. A full physical including rectal and/or pelvic exam should be performed to rule out the differential diagnoses. [Heinly AP: Irritable bowel syndrome, in Moser RL (ed): *Primary Care for Physician Assistants.* New York, McGraw-Hill, 1998, chap 6–17.]

6-46. **The correct answer is A.** The first goal of therapy is to normalize bowel habits. The best way to achieve this goal is with a high-fiber diet, adequate fluid intake, and regular exercise. These things all help the colon propel stool through the system with the mini-mum of stress, avoiding cramps, constipation, or diarrhea. [Heinly AP: Irritable bowel syndrome, in Moser RL (ed): *Primary Care for Physician Assistants.* New York, McGraw-Hill, 1998, chap 6–17.]

6-47. **The correct answer is A.** Given the long-standing diagnosis of IBS and the recent change in environment, it is tempting to take any of the other choices. But the correct action is to investigate the change. Since this patient's IBS has been stable until recently, you should look for the reason for a change. At her age, colon cancer, diverticulosis, or infectious colitis are all possibilities. Don't ignore changes; look for the cause and breathe easier if everything is negative. [Heinly AP: Irritable bowel syndrome, in Moser RL (ed): *Primary Care for Physician Assistants.* New York, McGraw-Hill, 1998, chap 6–17.]

6-48. **The correct answer is B.** Paradoxical diarrhea often is the presenting problem with underlying fecal impaction as the result of liquid stool leaking around the fecal mass. This is a particularly common presentation of fecal impaction in the institutionalized and in those with dementia or psychosis. Typical symptoms include anorexia, nausea, vomiting, and generalized, but not localized, abdominal pain. Rectal bleeding is not associated with fecal impaction, except in the rare instances where impaction is associated with colon perforation. [Wrenn K: Fecal impaction. *New Engl J Med* 321(10):658–662, 1989; Segal-Gidan F: Fecal impaction, in Moser RL (ed): *Primary Care for Physician Assistants*. New York, McGraw-Hill, 1998, chap 6–9.]

6-49. **The correct answer is D.** Most commonly, fecal impactions occur in the distal colon, particularly in individuals with decreased cognition or neurodegenerative disorders such as Alzheimer's, stroke, or multiple sclerosis. An impaction in the proximal colon should increase suspicion for underlying obstructive lesion, such as adenocarcinoma. A first-time impaction in the proximal colon warrants a more aggressive evaluation, including colonoscopy, than a distal impaction. [Wrenn K: Fecal impaction. *New Engl J Med* 321(10):658–662, 1989; Segal-Gidan F: Fecal impaction, in Moser RL (ed): *Primary Care for Physician Assistants*. New York, McGraw-Hill, 1998, chap 6–9.]

6-50. **The correct answer is A.** Enemas and suppositories alone may eliminate an impaction, but often do not. A mineral oil enema provides lubrication that can aid in removal of a fecal impaction. It is usually given after manual disimpaction has been done to begin to break up the fecal mass and stimulate the rectum for expulsion. Irritant laxatives and soap and hot water enemas should never be used as these irritate the rectal mucosa and may cause bleeding. [Wrenn K: Fecal impaction. *New Engl J Med* 321(10):658–662, 1989; Segal-Gidan F: Fecal impaction, in Moser RL (ed): *Primary Care for Physician Assistants*. New York, McGraw-Hill, 1998, chap 6–9.]

6-51. **The correct answer is E.** Native Americans are at high risk of gallbladder disease and cancer. In other populations, 4F's (female, fat, forty, and fertile) is the norm. Native American females may have cholelithiasis in their teens. Stones are quite rare in the Far East and Africa. Cholelithiasis increases with aging without sex specificity. [Heinly AP: Gallbladder disease, in Moser RL (ed): *Primary Care for Physician Assistants*. New York, McGraw-Hill, 1998, chap 6–10.]

6-52. **The correct answer is C.** Ceftriaxone can cause ceftriaxone-calcium sludge and may present as a cholelithiasis. The sludge occurs with recurrent use of ceftriaxone and is not commonly seen with a single injection. The cholelithiasis resolves with the discontinuation of the medication. [Heinly AP: Gallbladder disease, in Moser RL (ed): *Primary Care for Physician Assistants*. New York, McGraw-Hill, 1998, chap 6–10.]

6-53. **The correct answer is C.** This is the classic presentation of symptomatic cholelithiasis. The other choices are all potential differential diagnoses. Hepatitis would more commonly present with jaundice and hepatomegaly with generalized tenderness. Pancreatitis is ordinarily more epigastric to left upper quadrant pain radiating to the back with fever, nausea, and vomiting. Lactose intolerance causes abdominal cramping with profuse watery diarrhea. Peptic ulcer disease does not commonly radiate to the shoulders and is relieved with food. The abdominal tenderness is frequently found in the epigastrium. [Heinly AP: Gallbladder disease, in Moser RL (ed): *Primary Care for Physician Assistants*. New York, McGraw-Hill, 1998, chap 6–10.]

6-54. **The correct answer is B.** Approximately 40 to 50 percent of all adult AGE cases are caused by short-lived, food-borne bacteria. The rotaviruses are more common in children. Most infections are self-limiting and only need supportive care. Magnesium-based medications like antacids may cause a diarrhea state similar to AGE. *Clostridium diffi-*

cile is a food-borne pathogen that causes severe colitis and requires antibiotic therapy. Hyperthyroidism may cause a chronic diarrhea because of increased intestinal motility. [Heinly AP: Acute gastroenteritis, in Moser RL (ed): *Primary Care for Physician Assistants*. New York, McGraw-Hill, 1998, chap 6–1.]

6-55.   The correct answer is B.   Viral infections have been linked to specific raw oyster beds since the early 1990s. The other choices have been linked to bacterial infections: *Cyclospora* in strawberries; *Salmonella* in chicken, and *E. coli* in beef. Pork is most associated with trichinosis, which presents as an AGE. [Heinly AP: Acute gastroenteritis, in Moser RL (ed): *Primary Care for Physician Assistants*. New York, McGraw-Hill, 1998, chap 6–1.]

6-56.   The correct answer is C.   Given the patient's history, laboratory studies and radiographs are not warranted at this time. If symptoms persist over 48 h, then lab studies should be accomplished. If the patient is sent home, he should be sent home on a clear liquid diet that includes Pedialyte, Gatorade, or other sport drinks to replenish fluids and electrolytes. The *best option* is to get the patient started toward rehydration with 1 or 2 L of normal saline or Ringer's solution. Home instruction should include rest, pushing clear fluids (8 oz/h), and progress to bananas, rice, applesauce, toast (BRAT) diet as tolerated. Avoid all milk, cheese, or grease for 24 to 48 h. [Heinly AP: Acute gastroenteritis, in Moser RL (ed): *Primary Care for Physician Assistants*. New York, McGraw-Hill, 1998, chap 6–1.]

6-57.   The correct answer is E.   While the proper inspection and refrigeration of foods would decrease the cases of food-borne AGE, the best solution is good old-fashioned handwashing. The spread of AGE is primarily by oral-fecal route, good handwashing would help eliminate this connection. The use of prophylactic antibiotic or treatment of AGE with antibiotics is strongly discouraged. [Heinly AP: Acute gastroenteritis, in Moser RL (ed): *Primary Care for Physician Assistants*. New York, McGraw-Hill, 1998, chap 6–1.]

6-58.   The correct answer is C.   Life-style changes are the mainstay and should be the first line of therapy. GERD is a mechanical problem best controlled with small, well-chewed meals; a high-protein and low-fat diet; weight control and regular exercise; and elevation of the head of the bed 3 to 6 in. Medication therapy should be reserved for life-style change failures or persistent symptoms. Magnesium-based antacids cause diarrhea and should be avoided. [Heinly AP: Gastroesophageal reflux disease, in Moser RL (ed): *Primary Care for Physician Assistants*. New York, McGraw-Hill, 1998, chap 6–11.]

6-59.   The correct answer is C.   Omeprazole is a proton pump inhibitor, which with regular use can create a gastric achlorhydria. It is useful in the control of severe GERD because no acid production decreases the irritation the refluxant is able to cause. The yearly follow-up is required because prolonged periods of achlorhydria may predispose to gastric carcinoma or pernicious anemia. Aluminum-based antacids cause constipation and should be avoided. [Heinly AP: Gastroesophageal reflux disease, in Moser RL (ed): *Primary Care for Physician Assistants*. New York, McGraw-Hill, 1998, chap 6–11.]

6-60.   The correct answer is E.   A previous diagnosis of GERD does not impede a second look in the face of changing symptoms. This woman's life-style changes were apparently sufficient not to merit regular use of H_2 blockers or similar medications. The reappearance of symptoms at her age deserves an investigation. The absence of "red flag" symptoms such as weight loss, bleeding, or dysphagia precludes the need for an immediate EGD. [Heinly AP: Gastroesophageal reflux disease, in Moser RL (ed): *Primary Care for Physician Assistants*. New York, McGraw-Hill, 1998, chap 6–11.]

6-61.   The correct answer is D.   *Clostridium perfringens* is the most common source of food poisoning in the United States. It is generally self-limiting, causing profuse, watery diarrhea for 12 to 24 h. Of the other choices, *Campylobacter* and *Yersinia* are both associated with nausea, abdominal cramps, fever, and diarrhea. *H. capsulatum* and cytomegalovirus are seen in the immunocompromised patient with fever, abdominal pain, diarrhea, weight loss, and anorexia. [Heinly AP: Colitis, in Moser RL (ed): *Primary Care for Physician Assistants*. New York, McGraw-Hill, 1998, chap 6–4.]

6-62. The correct answer is E. Polyps may occur as singular or multiple lesions, and are usually less than or equal to 1 cm in diameter. Most polyps occur in the rectum or sigmoid colon. [Mayfield MS: Colorectal polyps, in Moser RL (ed): *Primary Care for Physician Assistants*. New York, McGraw-Hill, 1998, chap 6–5.]

6-63. The correct answer is C. There are few clinical findings associated with colorectal polyps. Polyps are generally not large enough to be palpable via the abdominal exam. GI bleeding that occurs is usually occult and emanates from the lower GI tract; therefore melena does not occur. Profuse rectal bleeding rarely occurs. [Mayfield MS: Colorectal polyps, in Moser RL (ed): *Primary Care for Physician Assistants*. New York, McGraw-Hill, 1998, chap 6–5.]

6-64. The correct answer is E. The most telling contrast between constipation and an acute abdominal event is the lack of systemic symptoms like fever, nausea, vomiting, or chills. The abdominal pain comes and goes in wavelike spasms without diaphoresis. The pain may be localized but frequently is generalized. Weight loss and tenesmus are not exclusive to a constipated state. [Heinly AP: Constipation, in Moser RL (ed): *Primary Care for Physician Assistants*. New York, McGraw-Hill, 1998, chap 6–6.]

6-65. The correct answer is A. With the absence of systemic symptoms, the plain films will most likely reveal gaseous distention of the colon with fecal material throughout the colon. With the exception of the EGD, the other tests may reveal constipation, but given the history would be unnecessarily costly and time consuming. [Heinly AP: Constipation, in Moser RL (ed): *Primary Care for Physician Assistants*. New York, McGraw-Hill, 1998, chap 6–6.]

6-66. The correct answer is A. There are very few medications that do not have the warning of constipation or diarrhea as a potential side effect. Some drug classes are known to have a higher risk of constipation, such as tricyclic antidepressants, narcotics, diuretics, and smooth-muscle relaxants. If these medications are used, a provision for constipation control should be made concurrently. [Heinly AP: Constipation, in Moser RL (ed): *Primary Care for Physician Assistants*. New York, McGraw-Hill, 1998, chap 6–6.]

6-67. The correct answer is D. Prophylaxis with antibiotics may be recommended for trips shorter than 2 weeks for the elderly or patients with GI or renal disease, cancer, or immunosuppression. Currently, trimethoprim-sulfamethoxazole once daily is recommended. The fluoroquinolones may be used as an alternative. Other recommendations include avoiding all freshwater sources such as ice cubes, fresh fruits and vegetables, and tap water (used for brushing teeth, drinking, etc.). Additionally, travelers should drink only commercially bottled beverages and eat only well-cooked foods that have not been rewarmed. [Heinly AP: Diarrhea, in Moser RL (ed): *Primary Care for Physician Assistants*. New York, McGraw-Hill, 1998, chap 6–7.]

6-68. The correct answer is D. Diarrhea is the most common gastrointestinal symptom of the immunocompromised patient. The initial stages may include a diarrhea state for 1 to 2 weeks. The patient with full-blown AIDS may experience multiple diarrhea states that are severe and recurrent due to the opportunistic nature of bowel flora. Bacteremia and sepsis are often seen and must be treated aggressively. The other choices can all cause diarrhea states, but they are seldom the presenting symptom. [Heinly AP: Diarrhea, in Moser RL (ed): *Primary Care for Physician Assistants*. New York, McGraw-Hill, 1998, chap 6–7.]

6-69.   The correct answer is C.   This is a classic presentation of diverticulosis. The pain is produced by colonic peristalsis, while there is increased intraluminal pressure. There is no inflammation, so systemic and peritoneal signs are absent. Renal colic, as a rule, is noted in the flank and lasts longer. IBS is not common to this age group and is generally associated with a diarrhea/constipation cycle. An ovarian cyst at this age would be unusual. Colon cancer is always a risk in this age group but the symptoms generally include a change in bowel habits and a dull, constant pain. [Heinly AP: Diverticular disease, in Moser RL (ed): *Primary Care for Physician Assistants.* New York, McGraw-Hill, 1998, chap 6–8.]

6-70.   The correct answer is D.   A barium study is considered the best way to define diverticulosis. The diverticuli appear as solitary lesions or in clumps of pedunculated mushroom-like appendages. The exam can also demonstrate paracolic abscesses, leaking diverticular sacs, fistulas, and stricture. The usefulness of a barium enema during acute diverticulitis is debated. Findings may be distorted by inflammation, and perforation is a risk. CT scan or ultrasound may be used as an alternative for acute diverticulitis. [Heinly AP: Diverticular disease, in Moser RL (ed): *Primary Care for Physician Assistants.* New York, McGraw-Hill, 1998, chap 6–8.]

6-71.   The correct answer is A.   The lack of esophageal peristalsis and the inability of the lower esophageal sphincter (LES) to open cause a progressive megaesophagus. The patient will experience some dysphagia, chest fullness or pain, weight loss, fatigue, and the inability to vomit. The other choices are good differential diagnoses. Distinguishing clues are the age and sex of the patient, cough, and the inability to vomit. As the esophagus fills with food there is inhalation of food into the bronchial tree causing a cough and frequent pneumonia or upper respiratory infection. Because of the tight LES tone, the patient cannot produce enough abdominal pressure to expel the contents through vomiting. [Heinly AP: Achalasia, in Moser RL (ed): *Primary Care for Physician Assistants.* New York, McGraw-Hill, 1998, chap 6–2.]

6-72.   The correct answer is C.   Femoral hernia is the likely diagnosis based on anatomic description in the superior aspect of the femoral triangle. These hernias account for 2 percent of groin hernias in men and one-third of groin hernias in women. The right side is more commonly affected than the left. These may be completely asymptomatic or can easily incarcerate or strangulate secondary to the narrow defect. The postsurgical recurrence rate is 5 to 10 percent. [Newell KA: Abdominal hernias, in Moser RL (ed): *Primary Care for Physician Assistants.* New York, McGraw-Hill, 1998, chap 6–24.]

6-73.   The correct answer is D.   Fecal stasis and fecalith formation is caused by small vegetable fibers obstructing the lumen. Hyperplasia of lymphoid follicles leads to obstruction of the lumen. Tumors, such as adenocarcinoma, can cause obstruction. [Jan PCH: Appendicitis, in Moser RL (ed): *Primary Care for Physician Assistants.* New York, McGraw-Hill, 1998, chap 6–26.]

6-74.   The correct answer is C.   Kehr's sign is usually associated with injury to the spleen. Psoas sign occurs when an inflamed appendix rests on the psoas and extension of the right thigh with resistance causes pain. Obturator sign is pain caused by flexion and extension of the thigh. Rovsing's sign is deep palpation of the left side to cause peritoneal irritation to the right side. [Jan PCH: Appendicitis, in Moser RL (ed): *Primary Care for Physician Assistants.* New York, McGraw-Hill, 1998, chap 6–26.]

6-75.   The correct answer is E.   *Entamoeba histolytica* is by far the most common amebiasis, causing colitis. It is found in the tropics and areas of poor sanitation. Symptoms develop 2 to 6 weeks after ingestion of the infectious cyst. Watery stools are frequent and of small volume associated with bleeding and mucus production. *Cryptosporidium* and *Isospora belli* may cause severe colitis in the immunocompromised patient. [Heinly AP: Colitis, in Moser RL (ed): *Primary Care for Physician Assistants.* New York, McGraw-Hill, 1998, chap 6–4.]

SECTION 7
HEMATOLOGY

7. HEMATOLOGY

QUESTIONS

DIRECTIONS: Each question below contains suggested responses. Choose the **one best** response to each question.

7-1. The blood count and differential on a person with thalassemia trait (minor) MOST often shows

(A) microcytic red blood cells
(B) normocytic red blood cells
(C) macrocytic red blood cells
(D) nucleated red blood cells

7-2. A 22-year-old asymptomatic black female had a routine complete blood count (CBC) that showed the following:

RBC count:	5.86	(normal 4.2–5.9 × 10⁶ μL)
Hgb:	11.2	(normal 12–16 g/dL)
Hct:	35.6	(normal 37–48%)
MVC:	74.4	(normal 86–98 fL)
RDW:	14.3	(normal 11.5–14.5%)

Subsequent iron studies yielded the following results:

serum iron:	98	(normal 50–175 μg/dL)
ferritin:	80	(normal 11–143 ng/mL)

The MOST likely diagnosis is

(A) iron-deficiency anemia
(B) thalassemia minor (trait)
(C) pernicious anemia
(D) folate deficiency

7-3. Which of the following is LEAST likely to present with a red blood cell profile of microcytosis?

(A) iron-deficiency anemia
(B) thalassemia major
(C) alcoholism
(D) lead poisoning

7-4. The thalassemias are caused by

(A) a defect in globin-chain synthesis
(B) a nuclear maturation defect
(C) an inflammatory suppressor of erythropoietin
(D) a nutritional deficiency

7-5. All of the following statements are TRUE regarding childhood leukemias EXCEPT

(A) The overall long-term survival rate in childhood is poor.
(B) The higher the WBC at diagnosis, the poorer the prognosis.
(C) The presence of CNS disease at diagnosis increases the likelihood of subsequent relapse.
(D) Children aged 2 through 10 have the best prognosis.

7-6. The MOST characteristic manifestation of Henoch-Schönlein purpura (HSP) is

(A) arthritis of the knee
(B) hematuria
(C) abdominal pain
(D) a typical rash

7-7. The treatment for Henoch-Schönlein purpura (HSP) is

(A) acyclovir
(B) a broad-spectrum antibiotic
(C) phlebotomy
(D) platelet transfusion
(E) none of the above

7-8. Increased iron absorption in the gut ("iron overload disease") is called

(A) aplastic
(B) erythropoiesis
(C) hemochromatosis
(D) pernicious
(E) polycythemia

7-9. What poses the BIGGEST risk of untreated hemochromatosis?

(A) increased skin pigmentation
(B) hepatomegaly
(C) blindness
(D) increased risk of hepatic malignancy
(E) leukemia

7-10. All of the following are signs and symptoms of hemochromatosis EXCEPT

(A) abdominal pain
(B) diabetes mellitus symptoms
(C) amenorrhea
(D) loss of libido or potency
(E) diarrhea

7-11. What is the BEST treatment for hereditary hemochromatosis?

(A) iron-free diet
(B) chelation therapy
(C) phlebotomy
(D) chemotherapy
(E) radiation therapy

7-12. All of the following have been implicated in the etiology of aplastic anemia EXCEPT

(A) smoking
(B) lindane
(C) fertilizers
(D) food additives
(E) chloramphenicol

7-13. Which of the following infectious diseases results in aplastic anemia in many cases?

(A) varicella
(B) influenza A
(C) hepatitis
(D) roseola
(E) streptococcal disease

7-14. All of the following statements regarding aplastic anemia are TRUE EXCEPT

(A) The onset is usually insidious.
(B) Patients are acutely ill-appearing with profound fatigue.
(C) Patients generally look and feel well.
(D) Patients often have infections exacerbated by neutropenia.
(E) Patients often have cutaneous bleeding associated with thrombocytopenia.

7-15. Although physical exam findings may be unremarkable in aplastic anemia, all of the following objective findings are possible EXCEPT

(A) ecchymoses/petechiae
(B) migratory arthralgias
(C) melena or occult stool blood
(D) retinal flame hemorrhage
(E) systolic ejection murmur

7-16. The serum ferritin level measures the

(A) plasma iron supply
(B) body iron stores
(C) red cell iron supply
(D) red cell turnover

7-17. The MOST common side effect of iron therapy is

(A) rash
(B) headaches
(C) gastrointestinal intolerance
(D) edema

7-18. A 50-year-old male is diagnosed with iron-deficiency anemia. The MOST important next step in management is

(A) dietary changes
(B) iron replacement therapy
(C) evaluation of the gastrointestinal tract
(D) evaluation of renal functioning

7-19. All of the following are expected signs or symptoms of severe iron-deficiency anemia EXCEPT

(A) pallor
(B) fatigue
(C) systolic murmur
(D) atrophic glossitis
(E) splenomegaly

7. HEMATOLOGY

ANSWERS

7-1. The correct answer is A. The thalassemias involve an inherited defect in hemoglobin synthesis that results in microcytic red blood cells. Marked microcytosis is common. [Deasy J: Thalassemia, in Moser RL (ed): *Primary Care for Physician Assistants*. New York, McGraw-Hill, 1998, chap 8–10.]

7-2. The correct answer is B. The mild anemia with relatively high RBC count with microcytosis and normal RDW suggest thalassemia. The normal iron and ferritin levels support the diagnosis. Pernicious anemia and folate deficiency are macrocytic anemias. In iron-deficiency anemia, the ferritin, and possibly also the serum iron, would be decreased. [Deasy J: Thalassemia, in Moser RL (ed): *Primary Care for Physician Assistants*. New York, McGraw-Hill, 1998, chap 8–10.]

7-3. The correct answer is C. An early sign of alcoholism is macrocytosis. Thalassemias, iron-deficiency anemia, and lead poisoning all result in microcytosis. [Deasy J: Thalassemia, in Moser RL (ed): *Primary Care for Physician Assistants*. New York, McGraw-Hill, 1998, chap 8–10.]

7-4. The correct answer is A. Thalassemias are caused by an inherited defect in globin-chain synthesis resulting in a cytoplasmic maturation defect. There is no relation to inflammation or diet. [Deasy J: Thalassemia, in Moser RL (ed): *Primary Care for Physician Assistants*. New York, McGraw-Hill, 1998, chap 8–10.]

7-5. The correct answer is A. The overall prognosis for childhood leukemias continues to improve, with 70 percent of patients achieving long-term disease-free survival. All of the other statements are true. [Wrigley DS: Leukemia, in Moser RL (ed): *Primary Care for Physician Assistants*. New York, McGraw-Hill, 1998, chap 8–2.]

7-6. The correct answer is D. The rash of HSP most typically occurs over the buttocks and lower extremities, but may involve the entire body. The skin lesions may consist of urticarial wheals, erythematous macules and papules, petechiae, and palpable purpura. [Deasy J: Henoch-Schönlein purpura, in Moser RL (ed): *Primary Care for Physician Assistants*. New York, McGraw-Hill, 1998, chap 8–7.]

7-7. The correct answer is E. There is no specific treatment for HSP. In severe cases, a short course of corticosteroids may provide relief of symptoms but does not alter the course of the disease. [Deasy J: Henoch-Schönlein purpura, in Moser RL (ed): *Primary Care for Physician Assistants*. New York, McGraw-Hill, 1998, chap 8–7.]

7-8. The correct answer is B. Hemochromatosis or "iron overload disease" is caused by increased iron absorption from the gut. Since the body cannot excrete iron, the excess iron is stored in organs such as the liver, pancreas, and heart. [Wrigley DS: Hemochromatosis, in Moser RL (ed): *Primary Care for Physician Assistants*. New York, McGraw-Hill, 1998, chap 8–5.]

7-9. The correct answer is D. The biggest risk of untreated hemochromatosis is the formation of hepatomas. Once established, the treatment of the disease does not affect the clinical outcome of the malignancy. Therefore, the goal is early identification and treatment, thereby reducing morbidity and mortality. [Wrigley DS: Hemochromatosis, in Moser RL (ed): *Primary Care for Physician Assistants*. New York, McGraw-Hill, 1998, chap 8–5.]

7-10. The correct answer is E. Diarrhea is a nonspecific symptom that is not commonly associated with hemochromatosis. All other choices are common signs and symptoms. Others include weakness, arthralgia, increased skin pigmentation, and hepatomegaly. [Wrigley DS: Hemochromatosis, in Moser RL (ed): *Primary Care for Physician Assistants*. New York, McGraw-Hill, 1998, chap 8–5.]

7-11. The correct answer is C. The best treatment is phlebotomy. One unit of blood conains 250 mg of iron, so at least 80 phlebotomies will be necessary to normalize total body iron. Once patients have achieved normal iron levels, then only 2 to 4 phlebotomies a year will be required for maintenance. Patients with induced (not hereditary) hemochromatosis associated with transfusion therapy should receive treatment with an iron-chelating agent. An iron-free diet is not necessary. [Wrigley DS: Hemochromatosis, in Moser RL (ed): *Primary Care for Physician Assistants*. New York, McGraw-Hill, 1998, chap 8–5.]

7-12. The correct answer is A. Smoking has not been directly implicated in the etiology of aplastic anemia. All of the other choices are among the numerous chemicals and drugs that can cause aplastic anemia. [Wrigley DS: Aplastic anemia, in Moser RL (ed): *Primary Care for Physician Assistants*. New York, McGraw-Hill, 1998, chap 8–4.]

7-13. The correct answer is C. Although many infectious diseases result in aplastic states, viral hepatitis commonly causes up to 5 percent of marrow failures, while Epstein-Barr, rubella, and parvo have also been implicated. [Wrigley DS: Aplastic anemia, in Moser RL (ed): *Primary Care for Physician Assistants*. New York, McGraw-Hill, 1998, chap 8–4.]

7-14. The correct answer is B. Except in severe, acquired cases, patients with aplastic anemia are not ill-appearing and do not have profound symptoms of anemia. Most patients have an insidious onset and generally look and feel well. [Wrigley DS: Aplastic anemia, in Moser RL (ed): *Primary Care for Physician Assistants*. New York, McGraw-Hill, 1998, chap 8–4.]

7-15. The correct answer is B. Migratory arthralgia is not associated with aplastic states; however, all the other choices may occur. Other objective findings include menorrhagia and purpura. [Wrigley DS: Aplastic anemia, in Moser RL (ed): *Primary Care for Physician Assistants*. New York, McGraw-Hill, 1998, chap 8–4.]

7-16. The correct answer is B. Ferritin is the major body iron-storage compound. A decrease in serum ferritin accompanies a decrease in tissue ferritin level, which reflects a decrease of body iron stores. Ferritin is currently the most sensitive test available for detection of iron deficiency. Ferritin may be falsely elevated in the presence of inflammation or infection. [Deasy J: Iron-deficiency anema, in Moser RL (ed): *Primary Care for Physician Assistants*. New York, McGraw-Hill, 1998, chap 8–1.]

7-17. The correct answer is C. At higher doses of iron, gastrointestinal intolerance, especially heartburn, nausea, and gastric discomfort can occur in as many as 50 percent of patients. Constipation and diarrhea also occur, but are less related to dose. Iron also turns stools black. [Deasy J: Iron-deficiency anema, in Moser RL (ed): *Primary Care for Physician Assistants*. New York, McGraw-Hill, 1998, chap 8–1.]

7-18. **The correct answer is C.** Iron-deficiency anemia is a symptom rather than a disease. The most important cause of IDA is blood loss, especially gastrointestinal blood loss. The presence of IDA in a 50-year-old male mandates a search for a potential source of gastrointestinal bleeding unless another cause is obvious. [Deasy J: Iron-deficiency anema, in Moser RL (ed): *Primary Care for Physician Assistants*. New York, McGraw-Hill, 1998, chap 8–1.]

7-19. **The corrct answer is E.** Splenomegaly is not an expected finding in iron-deficiency anemia. Its presence suggests another process is present. Pallor and fatigue and a systolic murmur are common to anemias. Severe iron deficiency causes skin and mucosal changes including a smooth tongue. [Deasy J: Iron-deficiency anema, in Moser RL (ed): *Primary Care for Physician Assistants*. New York, McGraw-Hill, 1998, chap 8–1.]

SECTION 8
INFECTIOUS DISEASE

8. INFECTIOUS DISEASE

QUESTIONS

DIRECTIONS: Each question below contains suggested responses. Choose the **one best** response to each question.

8-1. Which of the following statements about herpes zoster is TRUE?

(A) It is not contagious.
(B) Recurrences are common.
(C) Incidence increases with age.
(D) It is defined by a vesicular eruption.
(E) Topical therapy is of benefit.

8-2. Which of the following may be used to establish a definitive diagnosis of herpes simplex virus infection?

(A) acute antibody titer
(B) Tzanck smear
(C) Gram stain
(D) viral culture
(E) convalescent antibody titer

8-3. All of the following are appropriate for use in treating varicella EXCEPT

(A) systemic antihistamines
(B) oral acyclovir (Zovirax)
(C) calamine lotion
(D) aspirin
(E) cool baths

8-4. Which of the following statements about the varicella vaccine is TRUE?

(A) It is indicated in nonimmune pregnant women exposed to varicella.
(B) It confers lifelong immunity.
(C) It can be used to prevent zoster.
(D) A single dose between 12 and 18 months is recommended.
(E) It is of the dried-killed variety.

8-5. Varicella is MOST likely to occur in which of the following months?

(A) January
(B) April
(C) June
(D) August
(E) October

8-6. A normally healthy person who has resided in the agricultural San Joaquin Valley of California for the last 2 years comes to the office with complaints of fever, malaise, cough, and chest pain. The MOST likely differential for this illness would be

(A) histoplasmosis
(B) blastomycosis
(C) coccidioidomycosis
(D) aspergillosis

8-7. Coccidioidomycosis is a pathogen in infectious disease. The MOST common clinical presentation is as

(A) bronchitis
(B) meningitis
(C) osteomyelitis
(D) dermatitis

8-8. Treatment for cocci in a patient that shows signs or risks of dissemination is

(A) terconazole (Terazol)
(B) fluconazole (Diflucan)
(C) fulvicin (Griseofulvin)
(D) clotrimazole (Mycelex)

8-9. The MOST definite diagnostic test for active or current coccidioidomycosis is

(A) skin test
(B) serology titers
(C) spinal fluid analysis
(D) sputum culture

8-10. Which of the following is the causative organism of Lyme disease?

(A) *Leptospira*
(B) *Treponema*
(C) *Rickettsia typhi*
(D) *Rickettsia rickettsii*
(E) *Borrelia burgdorferi*

8-11. Which of the following areas has been relatively free of Lyme disease?

(A) Midwest
(B) Gulf Coast
(C) East Coast
(D) Pacific Coast
(E) the Great Lakes

8-12. Which of the following symptoms is usually the FIRST indication of the presence of Lyme disease?

(A) pruritus at the bite site
(B) cellulitis at the bite site
(C) erythema migrans
(D) fever and chills
(E) encephalopathy

8-13. A patient with stage 2 Lyme disease will MOST likely present with which of the following problems?

(A) Bell's palsy
(B) pneumonitis
(C) glomerulonephritis
(D) erythema nodosum
(E) palmar and sole rash

8-14. The predominant symptom in respiratory syncytial virus (RSV) that typically appears throughout the illness is

(A) pharyngitis
(B) cough
(C) sneezing
(D) rhinorrhea
(E) low-grade fever

8-15. What is the MOST efficient and reliable diagnostic test for RSV?

(A) immunofluorescent or enzyme staining
(B) sweat chloride test
(C) complete blood count
(D) routine culture
(E) chest x-ray

8-16. What is the MOST effective, current, and available therapy for treatment of severe RSV infections in children with congenital cardiopulmonary anomalies?

(A) vaccine (respiratory syncytial virus PFP)
(B) Ribavirin (hyperimmune RSV immunoglobulin G)
(C) interferon alfa-2a
(D) RSIVIG (RSV-neutralizing antibody/ respiratory syncytial immunoglobulin)
(E) maternal passive immunization

8-17. Which of the following is TRUE regarding diphtheria?

(A) The incidence of diphtheria has recently increased in the United States.
(B) The pseudomembrane extending to the bronchi is usually fatal.
(C) Neurologic symptoms are usually permanent.
(D) "Bull neck" refers to neck muscle spasms.
(E) Diphtheria has a long incubation period.

8-18. Unvaccinated diphtheria carriers should be treated with

(A) antitoxin
(B) antitoxin and antibiotics
(C) antibiotics
(D) diphtheria toxoid vaccination
(E) diphtheria toxoid vaccination and antibiotics

8-19. Rubella is also known as

(A) the brown measles
(B) the German measles
(C) the 7-day measles
(D) roseola
(E) all of the above

8-20. Which of the following is NOT a sign or symptom of rubella?

(A) erythematous rash
(B) suboccipital nodes
(C) polyarthralgia
(D) high fever
(E) malaise

8-21. Which of the following are the MOST common fatal complications of measles?

(A) fever and bacterial pneumonia
(B) croup and meningitis
(C) hepatitis and giant cell pneumonia
(D) meningitis and respiratory complications
(E) SSPE and immunodeficiency

8-22. Which of the following statements is TRUE regarding measles?

(A) An individual can recontract measles because the immunity conferred by an infection will decrease over time.

(B) A mother will pass measles immunity to her newborn only if she has had the natural disease.

(C) Measles temporarily depresses the humeral immune system.

(D) Less than half of patients contracting measles encephalitis survive without residual neurologic signs.

(E) Measles encephalitis is caused by a virus-produced neurotoxin.

8-23. Which of the following statements is TRUE regarding tetanus?

(A) All patients with contaminated wounds should be given a Td.

(B) HIV patients should avoid tetanus vaccines.

(C) Most cases of tetanus in the United States are preventable.

(D) Risus sardonicus is a condition where the jaw becomes locked.

(E) Dirty wounds should be infiltrated with tetanus immune globulin.

8-24. Which of the following is diagnostic of pertussis?

(A) lymphocytosis

(B) direct immunofluorescent assay (DFA) of nasopharyngeal secretions

(C) *Bordetella pertussis* cultured from nasopharyngeal specimens

(D) chest x-ray

(E) characteristic "whooping" cough is heard

8-25. Which of the following statements is TRUE regarding pertussis?

(A) Immunity from vaccination lasts about 3 years.

(B) Erythromycin will cure pertussis.

(C) Most adults are immune to pertussis.

(D) The risks of serious side effects from the vaccine are greater than morbidity and mortality risks from pertussis.

(E) The fatality rate of pertussis is 5 percent in the United States.

8-26. Which of the following statements about mumps is TRUE?

(A) Congenital mumps causes birth defects.

(B) As many as half of symptomatic mumps cases have cerebrospinal fluid pleocytosis.

(C) Infants should be immunized at 2, 4, and 6 months of age to prevent mumps.

(D) Mumps encephalitis carries a high morbidity and mortality.

(E) HIV is a contraindication to administration of mumps vaccine.

8-27. Which of the following is NOT a contraindication for mumps vaccination?

(A) young woman trying to get pregnant

(B) upper respiratory infection without fever

(C) pregnancy

(D) allergy to egg products

(E) immunodeficiency due to cancer chemotherapy

8-28. The etiologic agent of granuloma inguinale is

(A) *Haemophilus ducreyi*

(B) *Leishmania donovani*

(C) *Calymmatobacterium granulomatis*

(D) *Leptospira canicola*

8-29. Pharmacologic management for the treatment of granuloma inguinale includes

(A) ceftriaxone

(B) doxycycline

(C) vancomycin

(D) ampicillin

8-30. Complications of disseminated gonococcal infections include all EXCEPT

(A) septic arthritis

(B) aortic aneurysm

(C) myocarditis

(D) hepatitis

(E) meningitis

8-31. Risk factors for the development of an acute gonococcal salpingitis include all of the following EXCEPT

(A) presence of an IUD

(B) oral contraceptive usage

(C) previous STDs

(D) IV drug use

(E) HIV infection

8-32. The drug of choice for the treatment of chlamydial infections is

(A) amoxicillin
(B) ceftriaxone
(C) doxycycline
(D) penicillin
(E) spectinomycin

8-33. The MOST common clinical finding in female patients with chlamydial infection is a (an)

(A) asymptomatic patient, no evidence of infection present
(B) tender inguinal lymphadenopathy
(C) solitary ulcerated lesion
(D) purulent yellow-green discharge
(E) maculopapular lesion covering trunk and back

8-34. The drug of choice for the treatment of lympho-granuloma venereum (LGV) is

(A) erythromycin
(B) doxycycline
(C) spectinomycin
(D) ampicillin
(E) ceftriaxone

8-35. All of the following statements regarding LGV are TRUE EXCEPT

(A) A mucopurulent discharge is the most common clinical presentation.
(B) The etiologic agent is *Chlamydia trachomatis*.
(C) Regional lymph nodes undergo suppuration followed by extension into the adjacent tissues.
(D) Patients with LGV must have syphilis and herpes simplex virus (HSV) considered in the differential.
(E) Coinfection with other diseases is common in patients with genital ulcers.

8-36. All the following are signs and symptoms associated with toxic shock syndrome (TSS) EXCEPT

(A) desquamation of palms and soles 1 to 2 weeks after the illness
(B) diffuse macular rash
(C) hypertension
(D) temperature >38.9°C (102°F)
(E) vomiting

8-37. Which of the following is imperative in order to have a successful outcome in a patient with suspected TSS?

(A) abscess drainage
(B) aggressive supportive therapy including fluids, electrolyte, and blood product replacement
(C) identification of site of infection
(D) immediate removal of tampon
(E) starting an anti-staphylococcal antimicrobial agent

8-38. At which stage of syphilis are we likely to see condylomata lata?

(A) primary syphilis
(B) secondary syphilis
(C) latent syphilis
(D) tertiary syphilis

8-39. At which stage of syphilis is the patient likely to be asymptomatic?

(A) primary syphilis
(B) secondary syphilis
(C) latent syphilis
(D) tertiary syphilis

8-40. At which stage of syphilis are we likely to see an aortic aneurysm?

(A) primary syphilis
(B) secondary syphilis
(C) latent syphilis
(D) tertiary syphilis

8-41. Which of the following is LEAST likely to transmit the HIV virus?

(A) sharing of intravenous drug paraphernalia
(B) receptive anal intercourse with a condom
(C) breast milk
(D) saliva
(E) vaginal intercourse without a condom

8-42. The acute HIV syndrome MOST closely resembles

(A) influenza infection
(B) mononucleosis
(C) herpes zoster
(D) pityriasis rosea
(E) lymphoma

8-43. During the clinical latency of HIV disease

(A) the virus remains dormant
(B) the virus continues to replicate
(C) the immune system remains fully intact
(D) antigens become easily detectable

8-44. The MOST frequent manifestation of HIV disease following the acute syndrome is

(A) generalized lymphadenopathy
(B) fever and weight loss
(C) *Pneumocystis carinii* pneumonia
(D) Kaposi's sarcoma
(E) AIDS dementia

8-45. At what level CD4+ T helper cell count do the majority of HIV infected patients first start to exhibit manifestations of opportunistic infection?

(A) <50
(B) <100
(C) <200
(D) <300
(E) <500

8-46. The MOST serious side effect of treatment with ddI or ddC is

(A) myelosuppression
(B) nausea and vomiting
(C) chronic diarrhea
(D) taste disturbance
(E) pancreatitis

8-47. The MOST durable effects against HIV have been seen with

(A) Indinavir
(B) Invirase
(C) Nelfinavir
(D) Ritonavir
(E) AZT

8-48. The MOST common AIDS-defining illness in children less than 13 years old is

(A) Epstein-Barr infection
(B) gastroenteritis
(C) *Haemophilus influenzae*
(D) lymphoid interstitial pneumonia
(E) *Pneumocystis carinii* pneumonia

8-49. The TIS Classification for Kaposi's sarcoma (KS) is based on

(A) lymph node involvement, systemic symptoms, and fever
(B) number of lesions, biopsy characteristics, response to therapy
(C) number of lesions, locations, and visceral involvement
(D) tumor site(s), CD4+ count, systemic illness
(E) tumor size, CD4+ count, visceral involvement

8-50. Pulmonary KS is commonly mistakenly diagnosed as

(A) CMV pneumonia
(B) lymphoma
(C) *Pneumocystis carinii* pneumonia
(D) pneumococcus
(E) tuberculosis

8-51. Which of the following represents the MOST typical description of a KS lesion?

(A) brown to black tender nodule
(B) grouped, painful vesicles
(C) raised red to purple plaque
(D) red to purple blanching macule
(E) red to purple nonblanching macule

8-52. The MOST common neoplastic manifestation of HIV disease is

(A) adenocarcinoma
(B) Kaposi's sarcoma
(C) leukemia
(D) lymphoma
(E) melanoma

8-53. If a patient requests treatment for oral hairy leukoplakia you would recommend

(A) vigorous brushing and flossing daily to remove the lesion
(B) high-dose acyclovir
(C) AZT or another antiretroviral
(D) laser treatment
(E) cryotherapy

8-54. Oral hairy leukoplakia is

(A) infectious; kissing should be avoided until the lesion is treated
(B) premalignant; cytological scraping should be obtained every 3 months
(C) malignant; refer for immediate treatment
(D) indistinguishable from oral candidiasis
(E) a signal of advancing infection in HIV+ patients

8-55. The cause of oral hairy leukoplakia is

(A) smoking
(B) chewing tobacco
(C) Epstein-Barr virus
(D) HIV
(E) vitamin deficiency

8-56. The LEADING cause of meningitis in HIV+ patients is

(A) cryptococcus
(B) cytomegalovirus
(C) meningococcus
(D) toxoplasmosis
(E) tuberculosis

8-57. How is cryptococcus transmitted to humans?

(A) aerosolized particles from soil
(B) animal bites
(C) contaminated water
(D) human-to-human contact
(E) insect bites

8-58. Infection with *Cryptococcus neoformans* is manifested in HIV+ patients MOST commonly as

(A) cerebral cryptococcoma
(B) diarrhea
(C) meningitis
(D) pneumonia
(E) skin lesions

8-59. The MOST effective drug against cryptococcus is

(A) amphotericin B
(B) clotrimazole
(C) fluconazole
(D) ketoconazole
(E) zidovudine

8-60. After initial exposure to cytomegalovirus (CMV), a normal host will

(A) completely eradicate the virus
(B) continue to produce CMV IgM
(C) encapsulate the virus in selected lymph tissue
(D) recover but continue to harbor live virus
(E) remain virus-free until the immune system is stressed

8-61. Funduscopic changes typical of CMV retinitis include

(A) copper spots
(B) flame hemorrhages
(C) hyperpigmentation
(D) neovascularization
(E) white, cheesy exudates

8-62. Bone marrow suppression secondary to ganciclovir in the treatment of CMV is minimized by concurrent administration of

(A) interferon alpha
(B) erythropoietin
(C) foscarnet
(D) granulocyte-stimulating factor
(E) zidovudine

8-63. Infection with *Toxoplasma gondii* in an immunocompetent adult usually causes

(A) generalized papular rash
(B) encephalitis
(C) jaundice
(D) self-limited flulike symptoms
(E) no symptoms

8-64. *Toxoplasma gondii* is transmitted

(A) sexually
(B) in saliva
(C) through cooked, infected meat
(D) through contact with infected cat feces
(E) through household contact with an infected person

8-65. Congenital infection with *Toxoplasma gondii* can result in

(A) microcephalus
(B) jaundice
(C) hepatosplenomegaly
(D) mental retardation
(E) all of the above

8-66. To avoid toxoplasmosis, people with AIDS should

(A) give away all of their pets
(B) avoid contact with cat feces, and avoid ingesting raw meats and milk
(C) wear gloves when handling animals
(D) be immunized
(E) do nothing; HIV infection exists concurrently with toxoplasmosis

8-67. *Giardia lamblia* infection may be acquired by all of the following EXCEPT

(A) ingestion of contaminated food
(B) drinking contaminated water
(C) the bite of a mosquito
(D) fecal-oral transmission

8-68. Suspected infection with *Giardia lamblia* should be confirmed by ordering which of the following laboratory tests?

(A) complete blood count
(B) indirect hemagglutination test
(C) stool culture and sensitivities
(D) stool examination for ova and parasites

8-69. Which of the following is an appropriate treatment for *Giardia lamblia*?

(A) chloroquine
(B) metronidazole (Flagyl)
(C) amoxicillin
(D) praziquantel

8-70. Which of the following statements is TRUE regarding *Ascaris lumbricoides*?

(A) *A. lumbricoides* is transmitted sexually.
(B) *A. lumbricoides* is diagnosed by seeing cysts in a muscle biopsy.
(C) *A. lumbricoides* can cause pneumonia.
(D) The intermediate hosts of *A. lumbricoides* are dogs and cats.

8-71. Transmission of *Ascaris lumbricoides* is MOST often

(A) hand to mouth
(B) via contaminated food
(C) from an arthropod vector
(D) acquired sexually

8-72. Which is the MOST common bacterial food-borne pathogen in the United States?

(A) *Shigella sonnei*
(B) *Escherichia coli* O157:H7
(C) *Salmonella enteritidis*
(D) *Shigella dysenteriae*

8-73. Which of the following organisms requires notification of the lab for a special agar for identification?

(A) *Campylobacter jejuni*
(B) *Salmonella enteritidis*
(C) *Escherichia coli* O157:H7
(D) *Salmonella heidelberg*
(E) *Vibrio parahaemolyticus*

8-74. The MOST common symptom of pinworm infection is

(A) diarrhea
(B) abdominal pain
(C) perianal pruritus
(D) flatulence

8-75. The treatment for pinworms is

(A) metronidazole (Flagyl)
(B) Vermox
(C) chloroquine
(D) tetracycline

8-76. Which of the following BEST describes signs of elevating intracranial pressure?

(A) mental status changes, vomiting, and papilledema
(B) ataxia, positive Kernig's sign, and scalp tenderness with palpation
(C) nuchal rigidity, fever, and vomiting
(D) fever, forgetfulness, and nausea

8-77. A patient with a suspected brain abscess should undergo a search for

(A) a secondary source of infection located in the middle ear
(B) a potential secondary source of infection from a possibly infected tooth
(C) adequate views of the mastoids and sinuses
(D) an EEG study

8-78. The signs and symptoms of bacterial meningitis include all the following EXCEPT

(A) headache severe in character, constant, and in a generalized location
(B) a fixed dilated pupil associated with vomiting and fever
(C) drowsiness or coma
(D) irritability

8. INFECTIOUS DISEASE

ANSWERS

8-1. The correct answer is C. A distinct pattern of increasing incidence with increasing age exists, with two-thirds of patients over the age of 50. While patients with zoster do not spread the eruption of herpes zoster to other patients, it is communicable as varicella in nonimmune contacts. Recurrences do occur, but account for no more than 5 percent of all cases. Many disorders exhibit a vesicular eruption, and zoster may occur without any eruption. The only therapies shown to be of significant benefit are systemic. [Fenn WH: Herpes zoster, in Moser RL (ed): *Primary Care for Physician Assistants*. New York, McGraw-Hill, 1998, chap 2–17.]

8-2. The correct answer is D. Retrospective diagnosis by serologic studies requires both acute and convalescent titers. Gram staining is useful to distinguish simplex from such disorders as impetigo, but does not establish a viral etiology. Tzanck smears are useful to establish that a herpesvirus infection is present, but cannot identify herpes simplex specifically. [Fenn WH: Herpes simplex, in Moser RL (ed): *Primary Care for Physician Assistants*. New York, McGraw-Hill, 1998, chap 2–16.]

8-3. The correct answer is D. Aspirin is contraindicated during varicella due to the high risk of Reye's syndrome. Systemic antihistamines, calamine lotion, and cool baths are useful symptomatic therapies. Acyclovir (Zovirax) has been approved for use in varicella, but debate continues regarding its utility as a routine treatment. [Fenn WH: Varicella, in Moser RL (ed): *Primary Care for Physician Assistants*. New York, McGraw-Hill, 1998, chap 9–26.]

8-4. The correct answer is D. A single dose between 12 to 18 months is consistent with current CDC recommendations. Exposed nonimmune pregnant females should be treated with varicella-zoster immune globulin (VZIG). Data regarding duration of immunity and usefulness against zoster is still lacking. The currently approved vaccine is a live attenuated strain. [Fenn WH: Varicella, in Moser RL (ed): *Primary Care for Physician Assistants*. New York, McGraw-Hill, 1998, chap 9–26.]

8-5. The correct answer is C. Peak incidence of this disorder is late winter or early spring, and specifically the months of March through May. Why this occurs is unclear, but the pattern is distinct and well known. [Fenn WH: Varicella, in Moser RL (ed): *Primary Care for Physician Assistants*. New York, McGraw-Hill, 1998, chap 9–26.]

8-6. The correct answer is C. *Coccidioides immitis* is the fungus that resides in that geographic area. Healthy persons new to the area are most likely to contract the disease in the first 3 years of residency. Histoplasmosis would be more common in the mid-Atlantic and central parts of the United States. Blastomycosis is not common and would be found in the southeast, central, and mid-Atlantic states. Aspergillosis is more commonly found in patients that have <500 granulocyte count, have exposure to cytotoxic drugs, or are on large amounts of glucocorticoids. [Wrigley DS: Coccidioidomycosis, in Moser RL (ed): *Primary Care for Physician Assistants*. New York, McGraw-Hill, 1998, chap 9–7.]

8-7. The correct answer is A. *C. immitis* is a pathogen that is inhaled into the lungs and most commonly presents as a pulmonary infection. In certain individuals who are at risk, the disease may disseminate and cause a secondary complication of meningitis or osteomyelitis, as brain and bone are common sites of dissemination. Dermatitis is a cutaneous manifestation of pulmonary disease. [Wrigley DS: Coccidioidomycosis, in Moser RL (ed): *Primary Care for Physician Assistants*. New York, McGraw-Hill, 1998, chap 9–7.]

8-8. The correct answer is B. Fluconazole is currently the preferred "azole" of choice for those at risk of dissemination. Clinical trials have shown that it is better tolerated with fewer side effects than the other drugs in its group. Both clotrimazole and terconazole come in topical forms only, not oral, and therefore would not be treatments of choice for threatened systemic disease. Fulvicin has never been tried in clinical studies, probably because of poor GI absorption. [Wrigley DS: Coccidioidomycosis, in Moser RL (ed): *Primary Care for Physician Assistants*. New York, McGraw-Hill, 1998, chap 9–7.]

8-9. The correct answer is B. Serology titers give both the early response to infection, the IgM antibodies or Tube precipitin positive and/or they may give quantitation of IgG antibodies, representing infection longer than 30 days. A positive serology indicates active disease. A positive skin test is evident after 4 to 6 weeks of infection. It does not tell you when the person was exposed to the fungus. There are many people with positive valley fever skin tests that have never had symptoms. Approximately one-half of the residents in an endemic area are skin-test positive after 3 years or more of residency. Spinal fluid analysis will only show cocci in disseminated cases. Sputum cultures many times do not grow out the *C. immitis* fungus even with active disease present. [Wrigley DS: Coccidioidomycosis, in Moser RL (ed): *Primary Care for Physician Assistants*. New York, McGraw-Hill, 1998, chap 9–7.]

8-10. The correct answer is E. *B. burgdorferi* is the spirochete responsible for Lyme disease. The spirochete is carried to the human by the vector of deer ticks. [Heinly AP: Lyme disease, in Moser RL (ed): *Primary Care for Physician Assistants*. New York, McGraw-Hill, 1998, chap 9–3.]

8-11. The correct answer is B. The infected deer tick that carries the *B. burgdorferi* spirochete is common to the East and Midwest including the Great Lakes. The Western black-legged tick is common to the Pacific coast. As the deer population enlarges, Lyme disease may come to be seen nationwide. [Heinly AP: Lyme disease, in Moser RL (ed): *Primary Care for Physician Assistants*. New York, McGraw-Hill, 1998, chap 9–3.]

8-12. The correct answer is C. Fully 50 percent of all patients will experience the rash of Lyme disease, erythema migrans. Stage 1 of the disease is accompanied by the red, raised plaquelike annular lesion that enlarges over 3 to 4 weeks with central clearing. Patients may experience systemic symptoms resembling a viral illness with fever and headache. [Heinly AP: Lyme disease, in Moser RL (ed): *Primary Care for Physician Assistants*. New York, McGraw-Hill, 1998, chap 9–3.]

8-13. The correct answer is A. Cranial neuropathies, particularly facial neuropathies, are quite common in stage 2 of Lyme disease. The neuropathies may be painful and can last up to 6 to 8 months. Peripheral neuropathies are manifested with intermittent burning paresthesias and weakness. [Heinly AP: Lyme disease, in Moser RL (ed): *Primary Care for Physician Assistants*. New York, McGraw-Hill, 1998, chap 9–3.]

8-14. The correct answer is D. Rhinorrhea appears throughout the illness followed symptomatically by pharyngitis. They are the primary first signs of an infant infected with RSV. Within 1 to 3 days, a cough will start and may be associated with wheezing. A low-grade fever is a common but inconsistent sign. [van Deusen WJ: Respiratory syncytial virus, in Moser RL (ed): *Primary Care for Physician Assistants*. New York, McGraw-Hill, 1998, chap 9–20.]

8-15. **The correct answer is A.** The most efficient and expeditious means of diagnosing RSV is by obtaining a nasopharyngeal or throat swab sample for immunofluorescent or enzyme staining. It is 90 percent sensitive and specific for RSV infection. However, the standard of diagnosis remains with a routine culture, which can take 3 to 7 days. Routine lab tests are rarely helpful and are nonspecific. For example, a CBC typically shows a normal or elevated white and the differential can be shifted right or left. A standard PA and lateral chest x-ray may reveal peribronchial thickening (interstitial pneumonia) 50 to 80 percent of the time, hyperinflation/expansion 50 percent of the time, segmental consolidation 10 to 25 percent of the time, and airtrapping in 10 percent of the cases. Atelectasis and patchy infiltrates occur in many uncomplicated lower respiratory tract infections. A sweat chloride test is diagnostic for cystic fibrosis. [van Deusen WJ: Respiratory syncytial virus, in Moser RL (ed): *Primary Care for Physician Assistants.* New York, McGraw-Hill, 1998, chap 9–20.]

8-16. **The correct answer is B.** Aerosolized Ribavirin has been proven safe and effective in over 100,000 clinical test cases. It is expensive and should be reserved for and routinely administered to infants and children with underlying cardiopulmonary anomalies who are currently infected with RSV. RSIVIG (RSV-neutralizing antibody/respiratory syncytial immunoglobulin) is currently being used, but its benefits are still being tested. However, its use as prophylaxis for high-risk patients has proven beneficial. The RSV vaccine is currently being tested in children in phases of decreasing chronological age and offers hope in the future for all infants and children. Alpha-2A-interferon has been disappointing overall; however, administration in an aerosolized form is currently being tested. Maternal passive immunization is still in early trials. Although it has been proven safe for pregnant women, its benefit to the infant and child with RSV is unknown. [van Deusen WJ: Respiratory syncytial virus, in Moser RL (ed): *Primary Care for Physician Assistants.* New York, McGraw-Hill, 1998, chap 9–20.]

8-17. **The correct answer is B.** The pseudomembrane of diphtheria, when it extends to the bronchi, is usually fatal. The other responses are incorrect statements. [Dehn R: Diphtheria, in Moser RL (ed): *Primary Care for Physician Assistants.* New York, McGraw-Hill, 1998, chap 9–10.]

8-18. **The correct answer is E.** It is recommended that diphtheria carriers be treated both with antibiotics and the diphtheria toxoid vaccination. [Dehn R: Diphtheria, in Moser RL (ed): *Primary Care for Physician Assistants.* New York, McGraw-Hill, 1998, chap 9–10.]

8-19. **The correct answer is B.** Rubella is commonly known as the German measles, or the 3-day measles. It has also been called the easy measles, since the symptoms are quite mild. [Dehn R: Rubella, in Moser RL (ed): *Primary Care for Physician Assistants.* New York, McGraw-Hill, 1998, chap 9–21.]

8-20. **The correct answer is D.** High fevers are uncommon with rubella. The symptoms are quite mild, but occipital nodes, arthralgia, and a mild exanthemous rash can occur. [Dehn R: Rubella, in Moser RL (ed): *Primary Care for Physician Assistants.* New York, McGraw-Hill, 1998, chap 9–21.]

8-21. **The correct answer is D.** The most common fatal complications of measles are meningitis and respiratory complications, such as pneumonia. [Dehn R: Measles/Rubeola, in Moser RL (ed): *Primary Care for Physician Assistants.* New York, McGraw-Hill, 1998, chap 9–16.]

8-22. **The correct answer is D.** Measles encephalitis is a serious complication. Of the patients who survive, most will have some degree of residual neurologic signs. [Dehn R: Measles/Rubeola, in Moser RL (ed): *Primary Care for Physician Assistants.* New York, McGraw-Hill, 1998, chap 9–16.]

8-23. **The correct answer is C.** Tetanus is fully preventable by immunizations in the United States. [Dehn R: Tetanus, in Moser RL (ed): *Primary Care for Physician Assistants*. New York, McGraw-Hill, 1998, chap 9–23.]

8-24. **The correct answer is C.** *B. pertussis* cultured from nasopharyngeal specimens is diagnostic for the disease. [Dehn R: Pertussis, in Moser RL (ed): *Primary Care for Physician Assistants*. New York, McGraw-Hill, 1998, chap 9–18.]

8-25. **The correct answer is A.** Immunity from vaccination lasts about 3 years, so periodic reimmunization is required. [Dehn R: Pertussis, in Moser RL (ed): *Primary Care for Physician Assistants*. New York, McGraw-Hill, 1998, chap 9–18.]

8-26. **The correct answer is B.** As many as half of symptomatic mumps cases have CSF pleocytosis. This is the only true statement. [Dehn R: Mumps, in Moser RL (ed): *Primary Care for Physician Assistants*. New York, McGraw-Hill, 1998, chap 9–17.]

8-27. **The correct answer is B.** A mild nonfebrile upper respiratory infection is not a complication for immunization. The other statements are contraindications to the mumps vaccine. [Dehn R: Mumps, in Moser RL (ed): *Primary Care for Physician Assistants*. New York, McGraw-Hill, 1998, chap 9–17.]

8-28. **The correct answer is C.** *Calymmatobacterium granulomatis* is the etiologic agent of granuloma inguinale. The other organisms are responsible for diseases other than granuloma inguinale. [Hansen M: Granuloma inguinale, in Moser RL (ed): *Primary Care for Physician Assistants*. New York, McGraw-Hill, 1998, chap 9–14.]

8-29. **The correct answer is D.** Doxycycline is the drug of choice for the treatment of granuloma inguinale. [Hansen M: Granuloma inguinale, in Moser RL (ed): *Primary Care for Physician Assistants*. New York, McGraw-Hill, 1998, chap 9–14.]

8-30. **The correct answer is B.** An aortic aneurysm is more likely to be associated as a complication in the later stages of syphilis, not gonorrhea. The other choices have been associated in disseminated disease. [Hansen M: Gonorrhea, in Moser RL (ed): *Primary Care for Physician Assistants*. New York, McGraw-Hill, 1998, chap 9–13.]

8-31. **The correct answer is B.** The use of oral contraceptives is not a risk factor for acute gonococcal salpingitis. An IUD will increase the risk of pelvic imflammatory disease (PID). The presence or history of an STD is always a risk factor. Certain behaviors, such as substance abuse and IV drug use, are considered a risk factor. [Hansen M: Gonorrhea, in Moser RL (ed): *Primary Care for Physician Assistants*. New York, McGraw-Hill, 1998, chap 9–13.]

8-32. **The correct answer is C.** In a male or nonpregnant female, doxycycline remains the drug of choice for treating *Chlamydia*. [Hansen M: Chlamydia, in Moser RL (ed): *Primary Care for Physician Assistants*. New York, McGraw-Hill, 1998, chap 9–6.]

8-33. **The correct answer is A.** Chlamydial infections in women are usually asymptomatic. Even in males, the scanty, clear penile discharge is often ignored. [Hansen M: Chlamydia, in Moser RL (ed): *Primary Care for Physician Assistants*. New York, McGraw-Hill, 1998, chap 9–6.]

8-34. **The correct answer is B.** Doxycycline is the drug of choice for the treatment of LGV. [Hansen M: Lymphogranuloma venereum, in Moser RL (ed): *Primary Care for Physician Assistants*. New York, McGraw-Hill, 1998, chap 9–27.]

8-35. **The correct answer is A.** This is not a common clinical presentation of LGV. All other responses are true regarding LGV. [Hansen M: Lymphogranuloma venereum, in Moser RL (ed): *Primary Care for Physician Assistants.* New York, McGraw-Hill, 1998, chap 9–27.]

8-36. **The correct answer is C.** The onset is usually sudden, with high fever, watery diarrhea, and vomiting. An erythematous macular sunburn-like rash is seen over the face, proximal extremities, and trunk. Dehydration is evident, and the patient will have tachycardia and perhaps hypotension. Desquamation of palms and soles can occur 1 to 2 weeks after the illness wanes. [Julian TM et al (eds): *Appleton & Lange's Review of Obstetrics and Gynecology.* Norwalk, CT, Appleton & Lange, 1995.]

8-37. **The correct answer is B.** Although all of the responses are part of the treatment regimen for TSS, aggressive supportive therapy is imperative for a successful outcome. [Covino J: Toxic shock syndrome, in Moser RL (ed): *Primary Care for Physician Assistants.* New York, McGraw-Hill, 1998, chap 9–24.]

8-38. **The correct answer is B.** Condylomata lata is seen in the secondary stage of syphilis. [Hansen M: Syphilis, in Moser RL (ed): *Primary Care for Physician Assistants.* New York, McGraw-Hill, 1998, chap 9–22.]

8-39. **The correct answer is C.** The latent stage of syphilis is relatively free of syphilis-related symptoms. Primary syphilis has a chancre, the secondary stage has a characteristic rash, and the tertiary stage has numerous symptoms associated with the disease. [Hansen M: Syphilis, in Moser RL (ed): *Primary Care for Physician Assistants.* New York, McGraw-Hill, 1998, chap 9–22.]

8-40. **The correct answer is D.** Aortic aneurysms appear in the tertiary stages of syphilis. [Hansen M: Syphilis, in Moser RL (ed): *Primary Care for Physician Assistants.* New York, McGraw-Hill, 1998, chap 9–22.]

8-41. **The correct answer is D.** Transmission of HIV occurs mainly through sexual fluids and blood. There has never been any documented transmission of the virus through urine, saliva, tears, casual contact, respiratory droplets, or insects. [Cohen et al (eds): *The AIDS Knowledge Base: A Textbook on HIV Disease from the University of California at San Francisco and San Francisco General Hospital,* 2d ed. Boston, Little, Brown, 1994; Muma RD et al: *HIV Manual for Health Care Professionals,* 2d ed. Stamford, CT, Appleton & Lange, 1997; O'Connell CB: HIV/AIDS, in Moser RL (ed): *Primary Care for Physician Assistants.* New York, McGraw-Hill, 1998, chap 9–1.]

8-42. **The correct answer is B.** The acute HIV syndrome consists of lymphadenopathy with fever, pharyngitis, arthralgias, myalgias, headache, lethargy, and anorexia. It most closely resembles mononucleosis and, because of its perceived benign nature in presentation, is often missed or not reported. [Bennett JC, Plum F (eds): *Cecil Textbook of Medicine,* 20th ed. Philadelphia, Saunders, 1996; Fauci AS et al (eds): *Harrison's Principles of Internal Medicine,* 14th ed. New York, McGraw-Hill, 1998; Muma RD et al: *HIV Manual for Health Care Professionals,* 2d ed. Stamford, CT, Appleton & Lange, 1997; O'Connell CB: HIV/AIDS, in Moser RL (ed): *Primary Care for Physician Assistants.* New York, McGraw-Hill, 1998, chap 9–1.]

8-43. **The correct answer is B.** Although clinical symptoms may not become apparent for up to 10 years, the virus is very active, continuing to replicate and cause damage to the immune system. There is no true latent period. [Carmichael CG et al: *HIV/AIDS Primary Care Handbook.* Norwalk, CT, Appleton & Lange, 1995; O'Connell CB: HIV/AIDS, in Moser RL (ed): *Primary Care for Physician Assistants.* New York, McGraw-Hill, 1998, chap 9–1.]

8-44. The correct answer is A.   Generalized lymphadenopathy is encountered in the majority of cases of HIV infection, often present before the diagnosis of AIDS. [Muma RD et al: *HIV Manual for Health Care Professionals,* 2d ed. Stamford, CT, Appleton & Lange, 1997; Carmichael CG et al: *HIV/AIDS Primary Care Handbook.* Norwalk, CT, Appleton & Lange, 1995; Schacker T: Clinical and epidemiologic features of primary HIV infection. *Ann Intern Med* 125(4):257–264, 1996; O'Connell CB: HIV/AIDS, in Moser RL (ed): *Primary Care for Physician Assistants.* New York, McGraw-Hill, 1998, chap 9–1.]

8-45. The correct answer is C.   Most opportunistic infections, including *Pneumocystis carinii* pneumonia, the most common AIDS-defining illness in adults, manifest with a CD4+ count below 200. Many of the less common infections, including *Mycobacterium avium intracellulare,* are manifest at lower CD4+ cell counts. [Muma RD et al: *HIV Manual for Health Care Professionals,* 2d ed. Stamford, CT, Appleton & Lange, 1997; Carmichael CG et al: *HIV/AIDS Primary Care Handbook.* Norwalk, CT, Appleton & Lange, 1995; Schacker T: Clinical and epidemiologic features of primary HIV infection. *Ann Intern Med* 125(4):257–264, 1996; O'Connell CB: HIV/AIDS, in Moser RL (ed): *Primary Care for Physician Assistants.* New York, McGraw-Hill, 1998, chap 9–1.]

8-46. The correct answer is E.   Pancreatitis and peripheral neuropathy are the most serious side effects of ddl and ddC. Many practitioners will opt to analyze the amylase and lipase on a regular basis (every 1 to 2 months) in order to monitor for pancreatic inflammation. [Bartlett JC: *Pocketbook of Infectious Disease Therapy* (serial). Baltimore, Williams & Wilkins; O'Connell CB: HIV/AIDS, in Moser RL (ed): *Primary Care for Physician Assistants.* New York, McGraw-Hill, 1998, chap 9–1.]

8-47. The correct answer is A.   The most potent and the most durable effects against HIV have been seen with the three-drug combinations having Indinavir as the protease inhibitor (with AZT and another reverse transcriptase inhibitor). There have been reports of below-detection viral loads lasting for close to 2 years. More research will confirm this. [O'Connell CB: HIV/AIDS, in Moser RL (ed): *Primary Care for Physician Assistants.* New York, McGraw-Hill, 1998, chap 9–1.]

8-48. The correct answer is D.   Lymphoid interstitial pneumonia is very common in pediatric HIV+ patients. It is more common than *Pneumocystis* or any other bacterial or fungal infection. It is often the first indication of HIV infection. [Fauci AS, Braunwald E, Isselbacher KJ, et al (eds): *Harrison's Principles of Internal Medicine,* 14th ed. New York, McGraw-Hill, 1998; Bennett JC, Plum F (eds): *Cecil Textbook of Medicine,* 20th ed. Philadelphia, Saunders, 1996; O'Connell CB: HIV/AIDS, in Moser RL (ed): *Primary Care for Physician Assistants.* New York, McGraw-Hill, 1998, chap 9–1.]

8-49. The correct answer is D.   The National Institute of Allergy and Infectious Diseases AIDS Clinical Trials Group TIS Classification for Kaposi's sarcoma consists of tumor location and size, immune status (CD4+ count), and systemic illness (B symptoms, Karnofsky performance status, history of opportunistic infection, lymphoma, or thrush). The classification system is used as an indicator of prognosis and as a guide to choosing therapy. [Stone RM: Metastatic cancer of unknown primary site, in Fauci AS, Braunwald E, Isselbacher KJ, et al (eds): *Harrison's Principles of Internal Medicine,* 14th ed. New York, McGraw-Hill, 1998, chap 101; Bennett JC, Plum F (eds): *Cecil Textbook of Medicine,* 20th ed. Philadelphia, Saunders, 1996, p 1605.]

8-50. The correct answer is C.   Kaposi's sarcoma in the lung is fairly uncommon, but must be kept in mind whenever a patient who is HIV+ presents with dyspnea. KS commonly causes pleural effusions, but may appear without effusions. PCP remains the most common respiratory disease in HIV disease; failure to respond to PCP therapy should prompt the practitioner to search for other diagnoses, among them KS. [O'Connell CB: Kaposi's sarcoma, in Moser RL (ed): *Primary Care for Physician Assistants.* New York, McGraw-Hill, 1998, chap 9–2.]

8-51. The correct answer is D. Kaposi's sarcoma can appear in many forms, ranging from small macules to large plaques and nodules. The most common presentation, especially early in the disease, consists of small, violaceous, nonblanching cutaneous macules. [Bennett JC, Plum F (eds): *Cecil Textbook of Medicine,* 20th ed. Philadelphia, Saunders, 1996, p 1872; Fauci AS, Lane HC: Human immunodeficiency virus (HIV) disease: AIDS and related disorders, in Fauci AS, Braunwald E, Isselbacher KJ, et al (eds): *Harrison's Principles of Internal Medicine,* 14th ed. New York, McGraw-Hill, 1998, chap 308.]

8-52. The correct answer is B. Lymphoma, especially of the brain, is fairly common in advanced HIV disease. Kaposi's sarcoma is quite frequent. In the 1980s, KS was diagnosed at presentation in 40 percent of all HIV+ patients; today it is diagnosed in about 15 percent. [Bennett JC, Plum F (eds): *Cecil Textbook of Medicine,* 20th ed. Philadelphia, Saunders, 1996, p 1872.]

8-53. The correct answer is B. Antiretrovirals have not been shown to prevent or treat oral hairy leukoplakia (OHL). The lesions cannot be removed by brushing or flossing. Laser and cryotherapies are not used in the treatment of OHL. [O'Connell CB: HIV/AIDS, in Moser RL (ed): *Primary Care for Physician Assistants.* New York, McGraw-Hill, 1998, chap 9–1.]

8-54. The correct answer is E. Oral hairy leukoplakia is neither premalignant nor malignant; nor is it infectious. It is distinguished from oral candidiasis (thrush) by its lack of symptoms and the inability to remove it with gentle local scraping. [O'Connell CB: HIV/AIDS, in Moser RL (ed): *Primary Care for Physician Assistants.* New York, McGraw-Hill, 1998, chap 9–1.]

8-55. The correct answer is C. Although oral hairy leukoplakia is more frequently seen in smokers and in those with HIV, its cause is EBV. Vitamin deficiency and chewing tobacco are not known to be factors in growth of the lesion. [O'Connell CB: HIV/AIDS, in Moser RL (ed): *Primary Care for Physician Assistants.* New York, McGraw-Hill, 1998, chap 9–1.]

8-56. The correct answer is A. All of the pathogens listed can cause meningitis. In HIV+ patients, the most common pathogen responsible for meningitis is cryptococcus. [Fauci AS, Lane HC: Human immunodeficiency virus (HIV) disease: AIDS and related disorders, in Fauci AS, Braunwald E, Isselbacher KJ, et al (eds): *Harrison's Principles of Internal Medicine,* 14th ed. New York, McGraw-Hill, 1998, chap 308.]

8-57. The correct answer is A. Cryptococcus is endemic in pigeons and other birds and excreted in their droppings. The fungus remains in the soil and can be inhaled in aerosolized particles when the soil is disturbed. There is no evidence of human-to-human or animal (insect)-to-human transmission. [Dobkin JF: Opportunistic infections and AIDS. *Infect Med* 12(suppl A):65, 1995.]

8-58. The correct answer is C. Cryptococcal meningitis is the most common manifestation of cryptococcal infection, diagnosed in 67 to 85 percent of HIV+ patients with cryptococcal infection. A small percentage of these patients may develop cryptococcomas during their illness. Cryptococcal pneumonia is seen in about 40 percent of infected individuals and over 90 percent of these patients show concurrent meningeal infection with cryptococcus. [Fauci AS, Lane HC: Human immunodeficiency virus (HIV) disease: AIDS and related disorders, in Fauci AS, Braunwald E, Isselbacher KJ, et al (eds): *Harrison's Principles of Internal Medicine,* 14th ed. New York, McGraw-Hill, 1998, chap 308.]

8-59. The correct answer is A. In spite of its terrible reputation for side effects, amphotericin B remains the drug of choice against cryptococcus. It is more effective than any other antifungal therapy. Fluconazole is the first-choice alternative drug in patients unable to tolerate amphotericin B. The other azoles are less effective than fluconazole.

[Fauci AS, Lane HC: Human immunodeficiency virus (HIV) disease: AIDS and related disorders, in Fauci AS, Braunwald E, Isselbacher KJ, et al (eds): *Harrison's Principles of Internal Medicine,* 14th ed. New York, McGraw-Hill, 1998, chap 308.]

8-60. The correct answer is D. CMV remains in the body indefinitely, probably in multiple tissue sites as a latent virus. The virus is not eradicated when a person becomes immune compromised, so the virus is free to multiply and cause further disease. [Hirsch MS: Cytomegalovirus and human herpesvirus types 6, 7, and 8, in Fauci AS, Braunwald E, Isselbacher KJ, et al (eds): *Harrison's Principles of Internal Medicine,* 14th ed. New York, McGraw-Hill, 1998, chap 187; O'Connell CB: Cytomegalovirus infection, in Moser RL (ed): *Primary Care for Physician Assistants.* New York, McGraw-Hill, 1998, chap 9–9.]

8-61. The correct answer is E. White to yellow cheese-like exudates are the typical characteristics of CMV retinitis. [Bennet JC, Plum F (eds): *Cecil Textbook of Medicine,* 20th ed. Philadelphia, Saunders, 1996; O'Connell CB: Cytomegalovirus infection, in Moser RL (ed): *Primary Care for Physician Assistants.* New York, McGraw-Hill, 1998, chap 9–9.]

8-62. The correct answer is D. Granulocyte-stimulating factor is routinely given to patients being treated for CMV with ganciclovir to minimize leukopenia. Foscarnet is an alternative drug that does not cause bone marrow toxicity but can only be given to patients with normal renal function who can remain well hydrated. Zidovudine enhances the bone marrow toxicity of ganciclovir. [Fauci AS, Lane HC: Human immunodeficiency virus (HIV) disease: AIDS and related disorders, in Fauci AS, Braunwald E, Isselbacher KJ, et al (eds): *Harrison's Principles of Internal Medicine,* 14th ed. New York, McGraw-Hill, 1998, chap 308; O'Connell CB: Cytomegalovirus infection, in Moser RL (ed): *Primary Care for Physician Assistants.* New York, McGraw-Hill, 1998, chap 9–9.]

8-63. The correct answer is E. Rash, encephalitis, and jaundice may all be seen in infants who have been congenitally infected. Flulike symptoms may occur in pregnant women recently infected with toxoplasma. The typical immunocompetent adult suffers no symptoms at all. [Gallagher DM: Toxoplasmosis, in Moser RL (ed): *Primary Care for Physician Assistants.* New York, McGraw-Hill, 1998, chap 9–25.]

8-64. The correct answer is D. Cats are the definitive host of *T. gondii.* While cattle may harbor viable cysts, cooking the meat thoroughly would kill the parasite. Sexual, salivary, and household contacts are not modes of transmission. [Gallagher DM: Toxoplasmosis, in Moser RL (ed): *Primary Care for Physician Assistants.* New York, McGraw-Hill, 1998, chap 9–25.]

8-65. The correct answer is E. Congenital toxoplasmosis can result in a variety of serious conditions, including micro- and hydrocephaly, jaundice and hepatosplenomegaly, mental retardation, and cerebral calcifications. Congenital toxoplasmosis can also cause stillbirth. [Gallagher DM: Toxoplasmosis, in Moser RL (ed): *Primary Care for Physician Assistants.* New York, McGraw-Hill, 1998, chap 9–25.]

8-66. The correct answer is B. Since cats are the primary hosts of *T. gondii,* and cattle, goats, and poultry are intermediate hosts, viable oocysts can be transmitted if ingested. HIV and *T. gondii* are not transmitted by the same routes, so having one infection does not predispose the patient to having the other. There is no immunization against toxoplasma. [Gallagher DM: Toxoplasmosis, in Moser RL (ed): *Primary Care for Physician Assistants.* New York, McGraw-Hill, 1998, chap 9–25.]

8-67. The correct answer is C. The cyst is the infective stage and is transmitted fecally, orally, or through the ingestion of contaminated food or water. A vector, such as a mosquito, is not involved in transmission. [Deasy J: Giardiasis, in Moser RL (ed): *Primary Care for Physician Assistants.* New York, McGraw-Hill, 1998, chap 9–12.]

8-68.   The correct answer is D.   Microscopic examination of stools will usually reveal the cyst form of *Giardia lamblia* in semisolid or formed specimens and the trophozoite in liquid stools during the acute stage. [Deasy J: Giardiasis, in Moser RL (ed): *Primary Care for Physician Assistants.* New York, McGraw-Hill, 1998, chap 9–12.]

8-69.   The correct answer is B.   Metronidazole is the preferred drug in the treatment of *Giardia lamblia.* [Deasy J: Giardiasis, in Moser RL (ed): *Primary Care for Physician Assistants.* New York, McGraw-Hill, 1998, chap 9–12.]

8-70.   The correct answer is C.   Larval worms are carried via the bloodstream to the alveoli of the lungs, where they may cause pneumonia. Transmission is usually hand to mouth. The diagnosis is made by seeing the characteristic eggs in a stool sample. There is no intermediate host. [Deasy J: Ascariasis, in Moser RL (ed): *Primary Care for Physician Assistants.* New York, McGraw-Hill, 1998, chap 9–4.]

8-71.   The correct answer is A.   *Ascaris* eggs are deposited in the soil from feces and transmission usually occurs accidentally via the hand-to-mouth route. [Deasy J: Ascariasis, in Moser RL (ed): *Primary Care for Physician Assistants.* New York, McGraw-Hill, 1998, chap 9–4.]

8-72.   The correct answer is C.   *Salmonella enteritidis* is associated with consumption of raw or undercooked eggs, unpasteurized milk, and poultry products and is currently the most frequent cause of bacterial food-borne illness. [Davis R: Food-borne diseases, in Moser RL (ed): *Primary Care for Physician Assistants.* New York, McGraw-Hill, 1998, chap 9–30.]

8-73.   The correct answer is C.   *E. coli* O157:H7 requires a special agar that is different from routine stool cultures for enteric pathogens. The colonies are then assayed for the O157 antigen. [Davis R: Food-borne diseases, in Moser RL (ed): *Primary Care for Physician Assistants.* New York, McGraw-Hill, 1998, chap 9–30.]

8-74.   The correct answer is C.   The adult female migrates from the anus to deposit thousands of fertilized eggs on the perianal skin, resulting in pruritus. [Deasy J: Enterobiasis (Pinworms), in Moser RL (ed): *Primary Care for Physician Assistants.* New York, McGraw-Hill, 1998, chap 9–11.]

8-75.   The correct answer is B.   With its safety profile and ease of dosage, Vermox is the preferred treatment for pinworms. [Deasy J: Enterobiasis (Pinworms), in Moser RL (ed): *Primary Care for Physician Assistants.* New York, McGraw-Hill, 1998, chap 9–11.]

8-76.   The correct answer is A.   Changes in the mental status of a patient, vomiting, and papilledema are sure signs of increasing intracranial pressure, and need immediate evaluation as to the cause. [O'Brien-Norton M: Meningitis, in Moser RL (ed): *Primary Care for Physician Assistants.* New York, McGraw-Hill, 1998, chap 9–28.]

8-77.   The correct answer is C.   The source of the abscess is most likely the mastoid or paranasal sinuses, so adequate views of these structures are vital in detecting a brain abscess. [O'Brien-Norton M: Meningitis, in Moser RL (ed): *Primary Care for Physician Assistants.* New York, McGraw-Hill, 1998, chap 9–28.]

8-78.   The correct answer is B.   A fixed, dilated pupil associated with vomiting and fever is not a sign seen in meningitis. The other choices are seen in bacterial meningitis. [O'Brien-Norton M: Meningitis, in Moser RL (ed): *Primary Care for Physician Assistants.* New York, McGraw-Hill, 1998, chap 9–28.]

SECTION 9
MUSCULOSKELETAL

9. MUSCULOSKELETAL

QUESTIONS

DIRECTIONS: Each question below contains suggested responses. Choose the **one best** response to each question.

9-1. The MOST important patient history element to elicit in the evaluation of acute osteomyelitis is which of the following?

(A) family members that have had osteomyelitis
(B) contact with wild birds
(C) recent travel to foreign countries
(D) recent respiratory infection
(E) exposure to domestic animal feces

9-2. Which of the following is considered unreliable in the diagnosis and treatment of osteomyelitis?

(A) blood cultures
(B) bone and tissue histologic examination
(C) culture and sensitivity exam
(D) physical examination
(E) radiologic studies

9-3. MOST cases of osteomyelitis will manifest plain radiographic evidence of infection in what period of time after bacterial invasion of the bone?

(A) 2 to 3 days
(B) 2 to 4 weeks
(C) 4 to 6 months
(D) during first 24 h
(E) plain radiographs are not helpful and should not be performed

9-4. For the patient with penicillin allergy, the medication treatment of choice for acute staphylococci osteomyelitis might be

(A) gentamicin
(B) piperacillin
(C) clindamycin
(D) nafcillin
(E) cloxacillin

9-5. A 20-year-old male presents to your office complaining of pain and swelling in his right ankle and left knee. He also states he had a rash on his penis and dysuria 1 week ago that has disappeared. His MOST likely diagnosis is

(A) herpes simplex virus
(B) osteoarthritis
(C) rheumatoid arthritis
(D) Reiter's syndrome
(E) syphilis

9-6. The MOST common infectious organism isolated in patients with Reiter's syndrome is

(A) *Chlamydia trachomatis*
(B) *Neisseria gonorrhoeae*
(C) *Salmonella*
(D) *Shigella*
(E) *Ureaplasm urealyticum*

9-7. Patients with Reiter's syndrome usually present with all the following EXCEPT

(A) arthritis
(B) conjunctivitis
(C) hepatosplenomegaly
(D) mucopurulent cervicitis
(E) urethritis

9-8. Which of the following joints are NOT commonly involved in rheumatoid arthritis (RA)?

(A) sacroiliac
(B) knees
(C) metacarpophalangeal of hands
(D) wrists

9-9. Which of the following is NOT a characteristic deformity associated with rheumatoid arthritis (RA)?

(A) Swan-neck
(B) Boutonniere
(C) Heberden
(D) "Z"

9-10. What does a positive rheumatoid factor tell you of patients you suspect of having RA?

(A) They definitely have RA.
(B) They do not have RA.
(C) If they do have RA, they will have a more severe course.
(D) They have a lot of inflammation present.

9-11. Which of the following tests should be performed (and found normal) before starting a patient with rheumatoid arthritis on methotrexate (Rheumatrex) therapy?

(A) chest x-ray
(B) creatinine
(C) liver function studies and hepatitis B and C antibodies screen
(D) all of the above

9-12. Which of the following ethnic groups demonstrates the HIGHEST incidence of systemic lupus erythematosus (SLE)?

(A) African-Americans
(B) Caucasians
(C) Asians
(D) Native Americans
(E) Arabs

9-13. Which of the following is the MOST frequent cause of death in patients with SLE?

(A) renal disease
(B) cardiac disease
(C) pulmonary disease
(D) neurologic disease
(E) skeletal disease

9-14. An Apley's distraction test that causes pain at the medial aspect of the knee would indicate

(A) a torn medial collateral ligament
(B) a medial meniscus tear
(C) a popliteal tendon tear
(D) a torn medial retinaculum
(E) a quadriceps tendon tear

9-15. A history of a knee inversion injury while running in which a "pop" was felt and marked swelling occurred over a 10-min period would suggest which of the following injuries?

(A) a transverse fracture of the patella
(B) a torn lateral collateral ligament
(C) a torn anterior cruciate ligament
(D) a torn lateral meniscus
(E) a torn lateral retinaculum

9-16. Which of the following would be the MOST reliable historical indicator of a medial meniscus tear?

(A) pain
(B) swelling
(C) instability
(D) locking
(E) weakness

9-17. The MOST reliable historical indicator of a torn anterior cruciate ligament is

(A) pain
(B) swelling
(C) instability
(D) locking
(E) weakness

9-18. The MOST common chronic impairment and cause for disability for individuals under the age of 45 is

(A) low back problems
(B) heart disease
(C) hypertension
(D) diabetes mellitus

9-19. The MOST common cause for lower back pain is

(A) fracture
(B) primary spine tumors
(C) mechanical lumbar strain
(D) herniated lumbar disk

9-20. In the treatment of patients with acute low back pain, bed rest should be

(A) prescribed for most patients for a minimum of 2 days
(B) prescribed for most patients for a minimum of 4 days
(C) utilized primarily for patients with severe pain and limited to 4 days
(D) not utilized at all

9-21. A 19-year-old male presents with a 6-month history of gradual, intermittent back pain and morning stiffness that is improved with activity. Which of the following would be the MOST likely cause for these symptoms?

(A) polymyalgia rheumatica
(B) systemic lupus erythematosus
(C) rheumatoid arthritis
(D) ankylosing spondylitis

9-22. Disk herniations MOST commonly occur at the

(A) L4-L5 and L5-S1 levels
(B) L3-L4 and L4-L5 levels
(C) L2-L3 and L3-L4 levels
(D) L3-L4 and L5-S1 levels

9-23. A 65-year-old male presents with a 4-month history of lower back and bilateral extremity pain in the buttocks, legs, and thighs after prolonged walking and standing. He reports a gradual onset of these symptoms. He relates that his symptoms are relieved after 30 min of lying down in a supine position. Which of the following would MOST likely be the cause for his pain?

(A) rheumatoid arthritis
(B) ankylosing spondylitis
(C) mechanical back pain
(D) spinal stenosis

9-24. Which of the following statements is TRUE with regard to scaphoid fractures?

(A) Initial x-rays may be negative despite fracture.
(B) Treatment includes a thumb spica splint or cast for 4 to 6 weeks.
(C) Diagnosis and treatment is based on history and clinical findings (i.e., pain in anatomical snuffbox).
(D) Complications include development of avascular necrosis secondary to blood supply interruption.
(E) all of the above

9-25. A 24-year-old male presents to the emergency department the morning after an altercation in which he struck another person in the mouth with his fist. X-ray demonstrates fracture of the right fifth metacarpal neck with 50° of volar angulation. Which of the following is TRUE with regard to treatment?

(A) Careful examination of the metacarpophalangeal joint is mandatory prior to immobilization with an ulnar gutter splint.
(B) Ibuprofen may be helpful for analgesia.
(C) Elevation of the hand minimizes swelling and pain.
(D) Hematoma block may be helpful prior to attempting closed reduction.
(E) all of the above

9-26. A 22-year-old obese female presents with complaints of "left ankle pain" after stepping off a curb, excessively plantar flexing and inverting her ankle. Physical examination reveals swelling and joint tenderness over the base of the fifth metatarsal in addition to the lateral ankle. She has full range of motion at the ankle without pain. X-ray of the ankle is negative. However, avulsion fracture is noted at the fifth metatarsal on foot film. Which of the following statements is TRUE with regard to treatment?

(A) Hard-soled shoe is indicated for ambulation.
(B) Elevation minimizes swelling and pain.
(C) Application of ice at frequent intervals over the first 48 h minimizes swelling and pain.
(D) High clinical index of suspicion is warranted in this scenario so as not to miss a Jones fracture.
(E) all of the above

9-27. Physical exam findings consistent with the diagnosis of Osgood-Schlatter disease include all of the following EXCEPT

(A) anterior tibial tubercle swelling
(B) anterior tibial tubercle redness
(C) anterior tibial tubercle warmth
(D) anterior tibial tubercle pain
(E) increased knee pain with squatting

9-28. The examination or test that would be LEAST helpful in making a diagnosis of Osgood-Schlatter traction apophysitis is

(A) direct palpation
(B) Apley's compression or grind test
(C) stability testing of the medial and lateral collateral ligaments
(D) patella apprehension test
(E) AP and lateral radiographic views of the affected knee

9-29.   Which of the following is NOT a risk factor for the development of osteoarthritis (OA)?

(A)   increasing age
(B)   female gender
(C)   below normal weight
(D)   repetitive occupational joint use

9-30.   Which of the following characteristics is NOT common regarding the pain of OA?

(A)   aggravated with activity
(B)   alleviated with rest
(C)   described as a deep ache
(D)   bilateral

9-31.   Which of the following is pathognomonic for the diagnosis of OA?

(A)   Heberden's nodes
(B)   Bouchard's nodes
(C)   Scott's nodes
(D)   both A and B

9-32.   Which of the following is a criteria that must be present in addition to bilateral sacroiliitis to make the diagnosis of ankylosing spondylitis (AS)?

(A)   inflammatory back pain history
(B)   decreased range of motion of the lumbar spine
(C)   limited chest expansion
(D)   all of the above

9-33.   Which of the following is NOT considered to be a risk factor for the development of AS?

(A)   advancing age
(B)   male gender
(C)   family history

9-34.   Which of the following sacroiliac joint x-ray findings would NOT be consistent with the diagnosis of bilateral sacroiliitis?

(A)   blurring of the cortical margins
(B)   erosions
(C)   sclerosis
(D)   narrowing of the joint space

9-35.   The clinician must be aware of associated injury when evaluating a cervical strain/sprain. Which of the following is MOST commonly injured in cervical strain/sprain injury?

(A)   brain
(B)   globe of eye
(C)   larynx
(D)   lungs or trachea
(E)   heart or great vessels

9-36.   What factors are MOST important in the long-term care of the whiplash patient?

(A)   medications and periodic radiographic follow-up
(B)   patient education and psychological support
(C)   surgical correction pain syndrome
(D)   aggressive physical therapy on a short-term basis
(E)   intermittent muscle relaxer therapy in first month

9-37.   When difficulty evaluating C7 is encountered through normal radiographic positions in AP and lateral views, which of the following views may be MOST helpful in visualizing C7?

(A)   axillary view
(B)   open-mouth view
(C)   Swimmer's view
(D)   tangential cross-table view
(E)   hyperflexed view

9-38.   Injury to the sternocleidomastoid muscle on one side of the neck with associated swelling and muscle spasm can occur in acute neck injury and is termed

(A)   whiplash
(B)   torticollis
(C)   neck sprain
(D)   wryneck syndrome
(E)   radiculopathy

9-39.   Which of the following is diagnostic of gouty arthritis?

(A)   elevated serum uric acid
(B)   elevated sedimentation rate
(C)   rapid response to high-dose NSAIDs
(D)   urate crystals in the synovial fluid
(E)   calcium pyrophosphate dihydrate crystals in the synovial fluid

9-40.   The segment of the population at the HIGHEST risk for hip fracture is

(A)   elderly Caucasian women
(B)   elderly Caucasian men
(C)   elderly Hispanic women
(D)   elderly African-American women
(E)   elderly African-American men

9-41. Which of the following is the BEST study to confirm the diagnosis of a stress fracture of the hip in a 20-year-old runner?

(A) AP radiographs of the pelvis
(B) tomograms
(C) MRI
(D) scintigraphy
(E) CT

9-42. In a patient with a displaced femoral neck fracture, all of the following are indications for nonoperative treatment EXCEPT

(A) the presence of Parkinson's disease
(B) the presence of advanced arthritis
(C) physiological age over 70
(D) nonambulatory status before fracture
(E) pathologic fracture due to metastasis

9-43. A patient has sustained trauma to the great toe after dropping a 4-lb brick on his toe. His toe is diffusely swollen and red, and the nail is intact. Which of the following should be done FIRST?

(A) soak the toe in hot water
(B) order an x-ray to determine if a fracture is present
(C) put some bore holes through the nail to prevent a subungual hematoma
(D) wrap the toe tightly to prevent swelling
(E) provide an analgesic

9-44. What is the MOST likely life-threatening site of injury associated with a missed diagnosis or delayed treatment for Kawasaki disease (KD)?

(A) renal tubule
(B) coronary vascular/system vessels
(C) epidermis of the skin
(D) conjunctiva of the eyes
(E) large and small joints

9-45. What is the PRIMARY characteristic of the *acute phase* of Kawasaki disease?

(A) fever greater than 40°C (104°F) for at least 5 or more days
(B) irritability and altered mental status
(C) erythema and eruptions at toes, fingertips, palms, and soles
(D) systemic painful joint swelling and transient arthritis
(E) diarrhea, vomiting, and abdominal pain

9-46. All of the following need to be considered in the differential diagnosis of carpal tunnel syndrome EXCEPT

(A) C6-7 radiculopathy
(B) compression of the median nerve by an abnormal ligament of Struthers
(C) compression of the median nerve at Guyon's tunnel
(D) compression of the median nerve by the pronator teres
(E) thoracic outlet syndrome

9-47. The MOST common cause of carpal tunnel syndrome is

(A) pregnancy
(B) repetitive overuse
(C) rheumatoid arthritis
(D) diabetes mellitus
(E) hypothyroidism

9-48. Which of the following muscles is the MOST reliable to test for compression of the median nerve at the carpal tunnel?

(A) pronator teres
(B) flexor digitorum longus
(C) flexor pollicis brevis
(D) abductor pollicis brevis
(E) flexor carpi ulnaris

9-49. The conduction velocity of the median nerve in carpal tunnel syndrome is

(A) increased
(B) normal
(C) delayed
(D) dispersed
(E) stimulated

9-50. Which of the following is the correct position in which to splint the wrist of a patient with carpal tunnel syndrome?

(A) flexion
(B) extension
(C) pronation
(D) supination
(E) neutral

9. MUSCULOSKELETAL

ANSWERS

9-1. **The correct answer is D.** Respiratory infection or recent pharyngeal infection is often a precursor of osteomyelitis. There are not genetic markers or a positive correlation with family history. Contact with animals and travel to foreign countries have not been associated with an increased risk of osteomyelitis. [Cohen SM: Osteomyelitis, in Moser RL (ed): *Primary Care for Physician Assistants.* New York, McGraw-Hill, 1998, chap 10–17.]

9-2. **The correct answer is A.** Blood cultures have very low specificity and diagnostic accuracy in looking at the cause of osteomyelitis. While hematogenous spread of osteomyelitis is not uncommon, specifically identifying the organism of an infection from blood culture is only about 50 percent accurate when looking for treatment guidance. [Cohen SM: Osteomyelitis, in Moser RL (ed): *Primary Care for Physician Assistants.* New York, McGraw-Hill, 1998, chap 10–17.]

9-3. **The correct answer is B.** Radiographic evidence on plain films will manifest only after some bone destruction has occurred. In most cases this takes approximately 2 to 4 weeks to occur. Accurate determination of this effect is often confusing due to errors in estimating time from infection to visible radiographic damage. [Cohen SM: Osteomyelitis, in Moser RL (ed): *Primary Care for Physician Assistants.* New York, McGraw-Hill, 1998, chap 10–17.]

9-4. **The correct answer is C.** Clindamycin is the drug of choice in the uncomplicated patient. In the penicillin-allergic patient with staphylococcus osteomyelitis, the use of nafcillin and cloxacillin is contraindicated. Gentamicin is only recommended with the high-risk patient (e.g., IV drug user), and most often in combination with clindamycin. [Cohen SM: Osteomyelitis, in Moser RL (ed): *Primary Care for Physician Assistants.* New York, McGraw-Hill, 1998, chap 10–17.]

9-5. **The correct answer is D..** Reiter's syndrome is the most likely diagnosis in a young, sexually active male who presents with asymmetric arthritis and prior urologic complaints. [Covino JM: Reiter's syndrome, in Moser RL (ed): *Primary Care for Physician Assistants.* New York, McGraw-Hill, 1998, chap 10–9.]

9-6. **The correct answer is A.** *Chlamydia trachomatis* (serotypes D through K) is the most common infectious organism found in patients with Reiter's syndrome. It has been documented in approximately 50 percent of men with sexually acquired Reiter's syndrome. [Covino JM: Reiter's syndrome, in Moser RL (ed): *Primary Care for Physician Assistants.* New York, McGraw-Hill, 1998, chap 10–9.]

9-7. **The correct answer is C.** The diagnosis is straightforward in patients with arthritis, conjunctivitis, and urethritis/cervicitis. However, fewer than one-third of patients with Reiter's syndrome present with all three clinical findings. Mucocutaneous lesions occur in about 50 percent of patients. [Handsfield HH, Pollock PS: Arthritis associated with sexually transmitted diseases, in Holmes KK, Mårdh P-A-, Sparling PF, et al (eds): *Sexually Transmitted Diseases,* 2d ed. New York, McGraw-Hill, 1990, chap 61; Covino JM: Reiter's syndrome, in Moser RL (ed): *Primary Care for Physician Assistants.* New York, McGraw-Hill, 1998, chap 10–9.]

9-8. The correct answer is A. Rheumatoid arthritis (RA) generally affects the peripheral joints, not the axial joints. [Scott PM: Rheumatoid arthritis, in Moser RL (ed): *Primary Care for Physician Assistants.* New York, McGraw-Hill, 1998, chap 10–3.]

9-9. The correct answer is C. Heberden's nodes are characteristic of osteoarthritis, not rheumatoid arthritis. [Scott PM: Rheumatoid arthritis, in Moser RL (ed): *Primary Care for Physician Assistants.* New York, McGraw-Hill, 1998, chap 10–3.]

9-10. The correct answer is C. A positive RF does not confirm or exclude the diagnosis of RA. Additionally, it is not an indicator of inflammation. However, it is a useful prognostic test. [Scott PM: Rheumatoid arthritis, in Moser RL (ed): *Primary Care for Physician Assistants.* New York, McGraw-Hill, 1998, chap 10–3.]

9-11. The correct answer is D. Because of methotrexate's potential for hepatic, renal, and pulmonary complications, all of these tests should be performed and found normal. Additionally, the patient should have a normal CBC before instituting methotrexate therapy. The CBC, creatinine, and liver functions studies should be repeated at 1- to 2-month intervals while on methotrexate therapy. [Scott PM: Rheumatoid arthritis, in Moser RL (ed): *Primary Care for Physician Assistants.* New York, McGraw-Hill, 1998, chap 10–3.]

9-12. The correct answer is A. SLE affects members of all ethnic groups. However, in the United States the prevalence rate for African-American women is nearly three times the rate for Caucasian women. Certain Native American groups also have a somewhat higher occurrence rate than is found in the Caucasian population. [Mosier WA: Systemic lupus erythematosus, in Moser RL (ed): *Primary Care for Physician Assistants.* New York, McGraw-Hill, 1998, chap 10–10.]

9-13. The correct answer is A. Renal failure and heavy proteinuria are signs of a poor prognosis. The most frequent cause of death in patients with systemic lupus erythematosus is active renal disease. This is often accompanied by involvement of other organ systems. It also often occurs in conjunction with superimposed infection. [Mosier WA: Systemic lupus erythematosus, in Moser RL (ed): *Primary Care for Physician Assistants.* New York, McGraw-Hill, 1998, chap 10–10.]

9-14. The correct answer is A.. The Apley's distraction test is helpful in differentiating the source of medial joint-line pain. If the patient does not experience pain upon compression (meniscal tear), the examiner then stabilizes the thigh with one hand and pulls upward on the leg with the other. If the joint-line pain is due to an injury of the medial collateral ligament, pain will be elicited upon distraction. [Giles RS et al: Injuries of the knee, in Rockwood CA, Green DP (eds): *Fractures in Adults*, 4th ed. Philadelphia, Lippincott, 1996, vol 2, pp 2001–2126.]

9-15. The correct answer is C. The typical history obtained when an anterior cruciate ligament is torn is that of an inversion injury, followed by a pop that is heard or felt, and a massive, rapid effusion that is present within 5 to 10 min after the injury. [Giles RS et al: Injuries of the knee, in Rockwood CA, Green DP (eds): *Fractures in Adults*, 4th ed. Philadelphia, Lippincott, 1996, vol 2, pp 2001–2126.]

9-16. The correct answer is D. The most common cause of knee locking is a torn meniscus. When true locking occurs it is usually unexpected and the patient is unable to extend the knee past a given point. This is due to the torn portion of the meniscus extending into the joint and impinging between the femur and tibia. [Giles RS et al: Injuries of the knee, in Rockwood CA, Green DP (eds): *Fractures in Adults*, 4th ed. Philadelphia, Lippincott, 1996, vol 2, pp 2001–2126.]

9-17. The correct answer is C. Patients usually describe instability as "giving way" and, when present, it indicates injury to the primary and secondary stabilizers of the knee. Anterior cruciate ligament tears are noted by most patients to be symptomatic when pivoting is attempted. However, some may experience marked instability in straight-line walking. [Giles RS et al: Injuries of the knee, in Rockwood CA, Green DP (eds): *Fractures in Adults*, 4th ed. Philadelphia, Lippincott, 1996, vol 2, pp 2001–2126.]

9-18. The correct answer is A. Low back pain is a major cause of time and productivity loss at work. Surveys indicate that over 50 percent of working adults experience back pain yearly. In addition to lost work productivity, back problems affect an individual's quality of life by limiting their ability to participate in enjoyable activities. (US Department of Health and Human Services: Acute low back problems in adults: Assessment and treatment. *AHCPR Publication No. 95–06343*, 1994, p 1.)

9-19. The correct answer is C. Mechanical pain resulting from injuries to muscles, tendons, ligaments, deep fascia, disk, or bone accounts for the majority of back pain. Fractures and herniated lumbar disk etiologies are generally the result of trauma or a significant straining injury. Infections are most commonly associated with an invasive procedure. Primary spine tumors are rare. [Dunphy JE, Way LW, et al (eds): *Current Surgical Diagnosis and Treatment*. Los Altos, CA, Lange, 1994, p 1101.]

9-20. The correct answer is C. Newer studies indicate that for patients with acute low back pain, no bed rest and performance of normal activities as pain tolerates are superior to placing the patient on bed rest. Bed rest should be utilized for patients with severe limitations secondary to pain, and should be no more than 4 days. (US Department of Health and Human Services: Acute low back problems in adults: Assessment and treatment. *AHCPR Publication No. 95–06343*, 1994, p 13.)

9-21. The correct answer is D. Ankylosing spondylitis is a chronic systemic inflammatory disease of the joints and axial skeleton that commonly has an onset in the late teens or early twenties. It affects men more than women. The onset is gradual with intermittent exacerbations and back pain that radiates down the leg(s) posteriorly. Systemic lupus erythematosus and rheumatoid arthritis affect more women than men. Polymyalgia rheumatica commonly affects the elderly. [Tierney LM Jr, McPhee SJ, Papadakis MA (eds): *Current Medical Diagnosis and Treatment*. Los Altos, CA, Lange, 1996, p 755.]

9-22. The correct answer is A. The L4-L5 and L5-S1 levels are the sites of 95 percent of disk herniations. The majority of all clinically significant disk herniations producing lower extremity radiculopathy occur at these levels. Although not very specific, the straight leg raise test is a sensitive indicator for disk herniations at these levels. [Tierney LM Jr, McPhee SJ, Papadakis MA (eds): *Current Medical Diagnosis and Treatment*. Los Altos, CA, Lange, 1996, p 730.]

9-23. The correct answer is D. Spinal stenosis is a three-joint complex (disk and facet joints) condition that narrows the neural foramen, creating compression on the spinal cord. Most cases of stenosis are from degenerative changes of a collapsing disk and subsequent arthritis. The onset of symptoms is generally gradual and a common presentation is an elderly patient with nonspecific leg symptoms (neurogenic claudication). (US Department of Health and Human Services: Acute low back problems in adults: Assessment and treatment. *AHCPR Publication No. 95–06343*, 1994, p 20.)

9-24. The correct answer is E. Scaphoid fractures are diagnosed and treated based on history and clinical presentation. Initial x-rays are often read as negative. Repeat films at 2 weeks postinjury may be positive; however, many patients with fracture remain negative radiologically. Therefore, all patients with strong history and pain on anatomical snuffbox pressure are diagnosed and treated for fracture with thumb spica splint or cast for 4 to 6 weeks. Because the blood supply to the scaphoid is from distal to proximal, fracture at the middle portion (the most common location) interrupts this. These patients may develop avascular necrosis with chronic pain and mobility impairment. [Newell KA: Common fractures and dislocations, in Moser RL (ed): *Primary Care for Physician Assistants*. New York, McGraw-Hill, 1998, chap 10–2.]

9-25.   The correct answer is E.   All of the statements are true with regard to "boxer's fracture." Ibuprofen and elevation minimize swelling and pain. Hematoma block = 3 to 5 mL of plain 1% lidocaine can be injected into the fracture site prior to closed reduction to minimize volar angulation. Can accept 20° of volar angulation in fourth metacarpal and up to 40° in fifth metacarpal. Careful skin examination over the metacarpal phalangeal joint is critical to prevent "clenched-fist syndrome." This occurs as any opening of the skin over the joint may allow bacteria (often from oral flora considered a human bite) entry into the joint space. Once the laceration seals, the bacteria is trapped within. These injuries are often missed initially and the patient returns with splint intact complaining of increased pain and swelling at about 5 days postinjury. Removal of dressing and splint reveals a warm, red, swollen hand. Treatment usually requires hospital admission for IV antibiotics and surgical irrigation. [Newell KA: Common fractures and dislocations, in Moser RL (ed): *Primary Care for Physician Assistants*. New York, McGraw-Hill, 1998, chap 10–2.]

9-26.   The correct answer is E.   All of the statements are true. Note: Jones fracture is a transverse fracture of the fifth metatarsal often missed due to inadequate physical exam and x-ray views as the clinician attributes pain to an isolated ankle injury. The clinician sometimes fails to press over the base of the fifth metatarsal. If this pressing produces pain, then foot films should be obtained in addition to the ankle films. Jones fractures frequently develop nonunion or delayed union; therefore, a high clinical index of suspicion is necessary to correctly diagnose and appropriately treat (requires splint/cast, close orthopedic follow-up). [Newell KA: Common fractures and dislocations, in Moser RL (ed): *Primary Care for Physician Assistants*. New York, McGraw-Hill, 1998, chap 10–2.]

9-27.   The correct answer is C.   Patients with Osgood-Schlatter disease should not have warmth at the anterior tibial tubercle. Joint warmth is seen in conditions such as juvenile rheumatoid arthritis, septic arthritis, and osteomyelitis. Other findings not consistent with the diagnosis are medial or lateral knee tenderness, joint effusion, laxity in collateral or cruciate ligaments, and knee joint popping or clicking. Any one of these findings suggests other etiologies. Medial or lateral knee tenderness suggests collateral ligament injury. Meniscal tears may present with complaints of popping and/or clicking, especially with squatting or bending. Pain is increased at the anterior tibial tubercle with squatting in Osgood-Schlatter disease, but adventitious sounds are absent. [Pagels P: Osgood-Schlatter disease, in Moser RL (ed): *Primary Care for Physician Assistants*. New York, McGraw-Hill, 1998, chap 10–15.]

9-28.   The correct answer is E.   Following history and inspection, direct palpation of the knee is the most useful. In the case of Osgood-Schlatter disease the pain remains localized to the anterior tibial tubercle. The following provocative maneuvers are used to confirm that the pain is focal and not emanating from another source: Apley's grind test, used to diagnose a torn meniscus, is conducted with the patient prone and the affected knee flexed to 90°. Pressure is then placed on the heel during internal and external rotation, thus compressing the menisci between the tibia and femur. Meniscal damage probably exists if this maneuver is painful or produces popping or clicking. Stability testing for collateral ligament damage is accomplished by stressing the knee in valgus and palpating the medial joint line for pain and gapping. Reversing the procedure with varus stressing is used for the lateral collateral ligament. To rule out a patella prone to dislocation, the patella apprehension test is used. Have the patient lay supine with the knee in 30 to 45° of flexion with the quadriceps relaxed. Then apply pressure to the medial border of the patella, observing the patient for signs of apprehension (usually a loud plea to stop) as the patella begins to sublux. Since the diagnosis of traction apophysitis is made by history and direct physical exam, the radiograph is least useful. X-ray is employed primarily to rule out tumor or other bony abnormalities. If symptoms persist and activity is not modified, x-ray may reveal an enlarged irregular tibial tubercle, detached ossicles, or other soft tissue abnormalities. However, initial x-rays may show little, if any, changes. [Hoppenfeld S: *Physical Examination of the Spine and Extremities.* New York, Appleton, 1976, pp 171–196; Pagels P: Osgood-Schlatter disease, in Moser RL (ed): *Primary Care for Physician Assistants.* New York, McGraw-Hill, 1998, chap 10–15.]

9-29. The correct answer is C. Below-normal weight is a risk factor for osteoporosis, not osteoarthritis. The other three choices are proven risk factors for OA. [Scott PM: Osteoarthritis, in Moser RL (ed): *Primary Care for Physician Assistants.* New York, McGraw-Hill, 1998, chap 10–8.]

9-30. The correct answer is D. Although bilateral joint involvement is possible, unilateral pain is more characteristic in OA. Bilateral symptoms are seen more often with rheumatoid arthritis. [Scott PM: Osteoarthritis, in Moser RL (ed): *Primary Care for Physician Assistants.* New York, McGraw-Hill, 1998, chap 10–8.]

9-31. The correct answer is D. Heberden's and Bouchard's nodes, found in the DIPs and PIPs, respectively, are pathognomonic for osteoarthritis. Scott's nodes do not exist. [Scott PM: Osteoarthritis, in Moser RL (ed): *Primary Care for Physician Assistants.* New York, McGraw-Hill, 1998, chap 10–8.]

9-32. The correct answer is D. According to the modified New York criteria, any one of the above criteria plus radiographically confirmed sacroiliitis, is diagnostic for AS. [Scott PM: Ankylosing spondylitis, in Moser RL (ed): *Primary Care for Physician Assistants.* New York, McGraw-Hill, 1998, chap 10–4.]

9-33. The correct answer is A. The patient generally has the onset of symptoms in his/her late teens or early twenties. Onset after the age of 40 is rare. Male sex and family history are positively correlated with the development of AS. [Scott PM: Ankylosing spondylitis, in Moser RL (ed): *Primary Care for Physician Assistants.* New York, McGraw-Hill, 1998, chap 10–4.]

9-34. The correct answer is D. In sacroiliitis, the sacroiliac joint becomes "pseudo-widened" because of the erosions and sclerosis of the bony structures. [Scott PM: Osteoarthritis, in Moser RL (ed): *Primary Care for Physician Assistants.* New York, McGraw-Hill, 1998, chap 10–8.]

9-35. The correct answer is A. Cerebral contusion and concussion is the most common associated injury in whiplash. The forces that bring the neck into full extension and flexion causing soft tissue damage also are responsible for sending the brain forward and backward into the cranial vault. This injury can often cause symptoms and EEG changes. [Cohen SM: Cervical strain and sprain, in Moser RL (ed): *Primary Care for Physician Assistants.* New York, McGraw-Hill, 1998, chap 10–12.]

9-36. The correct answer is B. Patient education and psychological support are vital in the acute injury and chronic syndromes of whiplash. The emotional impact of this injury can be disabling and severe. Depression is an extremely common diagnosis in chronic neck pain syndromes after injury. Patient education supports patient understanding of self-care and treatment options. Medication should be regularly used in the acute phase of this injury and not on an as-needed basis. [Cohen SM: Cervical strain and sprain, in Moser RL (ed): *Primary Care for Physician Assistants.* New York, McGraw-Hill, 1998, chap 10–12.]

9-37. **The correct answer is C.** The Swimmer's view is ideal for visualizing the seventh cervical vertebrae. After visualization of C7-T1 has failed on a lateral C-spine radiograph, the Swimmer's view is often accomplished after repeat lateral radiographs with the shoulders pulled down manually. [Cohen SM: Cervical strain and sprain, in Moser RL (ed): *Primary Care for Physician Assistants*. New York, McGraw-Hill, 1998, chap 10–12.]

9-38. **The correct answer is B.** Torticollis is a muscle contraction or spasm that occurs idiopathically or after trauma. This most often occurs unilaterally. The patient presents with his/her head turned to the opposite side of the muscle contraction and a palpable band in the area of the sternocleidomastoid muscle. Neck sprain only occurs in ligament structures. Radiculopathy implies injury or compression to a nerve root and is associated with dermatomal symptom distribution. [Cohen SM: Cervical strain and sprain, in Moser RL (ed): *Primary Care for Physician Assistants*. New York, McGraw-Hill, 1998, chap 10–12.]

9-39. **The correct answer is D.** This is the most specific diagnostic test for gout. Elevated uric acid and ESR are nonspecific. [Dehn R: Gout, in Moser RL (ed): *Primary Care for Physician Assistants*. New York, McGraw-Hill, 1998, chap 10–5.]

9-40. **The correct answer is A.** Elderly Caucasian women are at twice the risk for hip fracture as compared with African-Americans and Hispanics and at 2.7 times the risk as compared to elderly Caucasian men. (Zinsmeister DE: The diagnosis and treatment of hip fractures. *J Am Acad Phys Assist* 6:542–551, 1993.)

9-41. **The correct answer is D.** Technetium 99m assists in the diagnosis of nondisplaced femoral neck stress fractures. The uptake of the radiopharmaceutical will demonstrate a stress fracture before the fracture will appear on conventional radiographs. (Zinsmeister DE: The diagnosis and treatment of hip fractures. *J Am Acad Phys Assist* 6:542–551, 1993.)

9-42. **The correct answer is D.** Operative treatment is generally considered the conservative option with relative contraindications limited to nonambulatory patients, severely demented patients in little pain, or those with life-threatening conditions who are at a high risk of death from anesthesia. (Zinsmeister DE: The diagnosis and treatment of hip fractures. *J Am Acad Phys Assist* 6:542–551, 1993.)

9-43. **The correct answer is B.** You should order an x-ray to determine if there is a fracture. The area should be soaked in cool water (never hot). If there is a subungual hematoma, it should be released to provide comfort for the patient, but prophylactic holes are not indicated. There is no need to wrap the toe tightly because this will cause increased pain. Elevation is important. A mild analgesic, such as acetaminophen, may be indicated. [Newell KA: Common fractures and dislocations, in Moser RL (ed): *Primary Care for Physician Assistants*. New York, McGraw-Hill, 1998, chap 10–2.]

9-44. **The correct answer is B.** Cardiac involvement is the predominant manifestation with missed or delayed diagnosis in Kawasaki disease, which includes vasculitis of the large coronary vessels. Epidermal skin changes and conjunctival changes are symptoms of KD; however, they do not have as potentially dangerous complications as the cardiac changes associated with a missed or delayed diagnosis. Systemic painful large and small joint swelling is a late phenomenon happening occasionally in older children. Penal tubular changes are not associated with this disease. [van Deusen WJ: Kawasaki disease, in Moser RL (ed): *Primary Care for Physician Assistants*. New York, McGraw-Hill, 1998, chap 10–6.]

9-45. **The correct answer is A.** High fever [over 40°C (104°F)] for at least 5 days occurs in the acute stage of Kawasaki disease (KD) and is the hallmark symptom. Erythema and eruptions at toes, fingertips and palms, and soles are significant in the diagnosis of KD but occur in the subacute phase. Children are typically irritable and may have altered mental status in a variety of illnesses. The more obscure symptoms of diarrhea, vomiting, and abdominal pain occur during the acute phase, but none of them is the primary characteristic symptom. [van Deusen WJ: Kawasaki disease, in Moser RL (ed): *Primary Care for Physician Assistants.* New York, McGraw-Hill, 1998, chap 10–6.]

9-46. The correct answer is C.   The ulnar nerve travels through Guyon's tunnel and compression will result in sensory symptoms in the ulnar aspect of the ring finger and small finger. Motor symptoms will appear in the hypothenar muscle group and adductors and abductors of the fingers. (Rosenbaum RB, Ochoa JL: *Carpal Tunnel Syndrome and Other Disorders of the Median Nerve.* Boston, Butterworth-Heinemann, 1993.)

9-47. The correct answer is B.   Repetitive overuse is the most common cause of carpal tunnel syndrome. Actions performed repetitively in the workplace or during leisure activities may result in swelling of the synovium or thickening of the transverse carpal ligament, which causes compression of the median nerve. (Rosenbaum RB, Ochoa JL, *Carpal Tunnel Syndrome and Other Disorders of the Median Nerve.* Boston, Butterworth-Heinemann, 1993.)

9-48. The correct answer is D.   Motor testing in carpal tunnel syndrome is normally limited to the abductor pollicis brevis since it is the least likely of the thenar muscles to receive innervation from the ulnar nerve and is the easiest to isolate. (Rosenbaum RB, Ochoa JL: *Carpal Tunnel Syndrome and Other Disorders of the Median Nerve. Boston,* Butterworth-Heinemann, 1993.)

9-49. The correct answer is C.   Conduction velocity is a direct measurement of the latency and records the time from stimulus to response. In carpal tunnel syndrome, conduction velocity will be delayed due to demyelination of median nerve fibers. (Rosenbaum RB, Ochoa JL: *Carpal Tunnel Syndrome and Other Disorders of the Median Nerve.* Boston, Butterworth-Heinemann, 1993.)

9-50. The correct answer is E.   When splinting the wrist of a patient with carpal tunnel syndrome, the wrist should be placed in the neutral position. If the wrist is flexed, the volume of the tunnel will be decreased and subject the nerve to further compression. If the wrist is placed in extension, the median nerve will be forced against the transverse carpal ligament. (Rosenbaum RB, Ochoa JL: *Carpal Tunnel Syndrome and Other Disorders of the Median Nerve.* Boston, Butterworth-Heinemann, 1993.)

SECTION 10
NEUROLOGY

10. NEUROLOGY

QUESTIONS

DIRECTIONS: Each question below contains suggested responses. Choose the **one best** response to each question.

10-1. The primary headache MOST likely to have a genetically linked base is

(A) migraine headache
(B) cluster headache
(C) atypical headache
(D) sinus headache

10-2. A primary goal of treatment of benign organic headache is

(A) complete eradication of the headache
(B) decrease functionality, frequency, and duration of headaches
(C) choosing the right analgesic
(D) ruling out an intracranial lesion with an MRI

10-3. All of the following are signs and symptoms that may indicate the need to perform additional tests or consult with a specialist EXCEPT

(A) pain severe enough to disturb sleep
(B) progressively worsening headaches
(C) pain relieved by nonprescription drugs
(D) neurologic abnormalities on examination

10-4. Diagnostic criteria for dementia require which of the following?

(A) memory loss
(B) functional loss
(C) memory loss and loss in one other cognitive domain
(D) memory loss, loss in one other cognitive area, and functional loss

10-5. Regarding dementia, routine mental status testing is

(A) useless, and should be reserved for those with a complaint of memory loss
(B) a good screening tool for early dementia
(C) difficult to accurately learn and use
(D) good for diagnosing the underlying etiology of a dementia

10-6. Routine laboratory screening for reversible or exacerbating conditions in a patient with a suspected dementia includes

(A) HIV testing
(B) thyroid function tests
(C) urine drug toxicity screen
(D) apo E lipoprotein

10-7. Normal-pressure hydrocephalus (NPH) presents with dementia and

(A) urinary incontinence and gait instability
(B) acute confusion
(C) nausea, vomiting, and other signs of increased intracranial pressure
(D) muscle incoordination and swallowing problems

10-8. A 68-year-old man is brought into the clinic with recent onset of confusion. Which of the following medications that you recently prescribed is the MOST likely cause or contributing factor?

(A) levothyroxine sodium (Synthroid)
(B) flurazepam
(C) nifedipine
(D) ranitidine

10-9. Which of the following is the GREATEST single risk factor for developing Alzheimer's disease?

(A) family history
(B) age
(C) female gender
(D) aluminum exposure

10-10. A diagnosis of definite Alzheimer's disease requires

(A) clinical diagnosis of dementia without any other known cause
(B) cortical atrophy by CT or MRI scan
(C) clinical diagnosis of dementia and pathologic specimen with tangles and plaques
(D) clinical diagnosis of dementia of no other known etiology and a family history of dementia in one first-degree relative

10-11. The definitive laboratory test for a clinical diagnosis of Alzheimer's disease is

(A) MRI of the brain
(B) PET or SPECT scan of the brain
(C) apo E genetic test
(D) none

10-12. The presence of which of the following is NOT consistent with a diagnosis of probable Alzheimer's disease?

(A) normal CT or MRI scan of the brain
(B) new-onset seizure disorder
(C) abnormal electroencephalogram (EEG)
(D) hypertension

10-13. The use of tacrine (Cognex) for the treatment of Alzheimer's disease

(A) is not proven and is considered experimental
(B) requires referral to a specialist
(C) requires frequent monitoring of liver enzymes
(D) is contraindicated in a patient on any other medication

10-14. Clinical features typical of Alzheimer's disease include

(A) global memory problems
(B) memory loss and language deterioration
(C) memory loss and vision impairment
(D) poor judgment

10-15. Which of the following is the MOST common idiopathic localization-related seizure disorder?

(A) benign childhood epilepsy with centrotemporal spikes (benign rolandic epilepsy)
(B) childhood epilepsy with occipital paroxysms
(C) chronic progressive epilepsia partialis continua of childhood (Kojewnikoff's epilepsy)
(D) benign neonatal familial convulsions
(E) temporal lobe epilepsies (amygdalopippocampal, lateral)

10-16. Which of the following is the MOST common type of nonconvulsive seizure?

(A) absence seizure
(B) myoclonic seizure
(C) clonic seizure
(D) tonic seizure
(E) atomic seizure

10-17. A patient is said to be in status epilepticus if their seizure lasts longer than which of the following?

(A) 5 min
(B) 10 min
(C) 20 min
(D) 30 min
(E) 40 min

10-18. Which of the following is the MOST commonly occurring demyelinating disease of the central nervous system?

(A) postinfectious encephalomyelitis
(B) postvaccinal encephalomyelitis
(C) acute necrotizing hemorrhagic encephalomyelitis
(D) adrenoleukodystrophy
(E) multiple sclerosis

10-19. Which of the following is a common sign of multiple sclerosis?

(A) abnormal eye movements
(B) macular degeneration
(C) retinal damage
(D) bilateral optic neuropathy
(E) abrupt loss of vision

10-20. Which of the following is the MOST typical age of onset for multiple sclerosis?

(A) birth to age 8
(B) ages 9 to 14
(C) ages 15 to 40
(D) ages 41 to 50
(E) ages 51 to 60

10-21. Which of the following is the area of pathologic focus of multiple sclerosis?

(A) myelin coating of nerve fibers
(B) meninges
(C) nerve roots
(D) lymphoid tissue
(E) cerebrospinal fluid

10-22. Which of the following is the basis for diagnosing multiple sclerosis?

(A) clinical findings
(B) electroencephalography
(C) computed tomography
(D) myelography
(E) evoked potential studies

10-23. Rigidity, tremor, bradykinesia, and postural instability are cardinal signs of

(A) Huntington's disease
(B) normal aging
(C) Guillain-Barré syndrome
(D) Parkinson's disease
(E) complex partial seizures

10-24. The pathologic hallmark of Parkinson's disease is considered to be

(A) nail pitting
(B) the Lewy body
(C) essential tremor
(D) postural instability
(E) no change in the globus pallidus

10-25. Which of the following medications is considered to be the basis for treatment of Parkinson's disease?

(A) carbidopa-levodopa (Sinemet)
(B) selegiline (Eldepryl)
(C) trihexyphenidyl (Artane)
(D) propranolol (Inderal)
(E) all are used in the treatment of Parkinson's disease

10-26. The etiology of myasthenia gravis is thought to be

(A) viral
(B) bacterial
(C) trauma
(D) autoimmune
(E) unknown

10-27. Most myasthenic patients initially present with the chief complaints of

(A) weakness and easy fatigability
(B) nausea and vomiting
(C) numbness and tingling
(D) pain and restlessness
(E) none of the above

10-28. The defect in myasthenia gravis that prohibits conduction of the action potential from the presynaptic membrane to the postsynaptic membrane is

(A) erosion of the myelin sheath
(B) decreased synthesis of acetylcholine
(C) decreased concentration of acetylcholine in the synapse
(D) destruction of acetylcholine receptor sites
(E) abnormally high levels of sodium ions

10-29. Which of the following cranial nerves mediates the reactions of nausea and vomiting?

(A) CN I
(B) CN X
(C) CN IX
(D) CN VII
(E) CN XII

10. NEUROLOGY

10-1. **The correct answer is A.** There are often strong family histories of migraine headaches. The other types of headaches are not felt to be genetically linked. [Weiss AG: Headaches, in Moser RL (ed): *Primary Care for Physician Assistants*. New York, McGraw-Hill, 1998, chap 11–3.]

10-2. **The correct answer is B.** Decreasing functionality, frequency, and duration of headaches are the primary goals of treatment. [Weiss AG: Headaches, in Moser RL (ed): *Primary Care for Physician Assistants*. New York, McGraw-Hill, 1998, chap 11–3.]

10-3. **The correct answer is C.** If pain is relieved by nonprescription drugs there is no need for additional tests or consultation with a specialist. Regardless of a patient's response to analgesics, additional tests may be indicated. The other signs and symptoms listed are indications for further evaluation. [Weiss AG: Headaches, in Moser RL (ed): *Primary Care for Physician Assistants*. New York, McGraw-Hill, 1998, chap 11–3.]

10-4. **The correct answer is D.** A diagnosis of dementia is more than memory loss alone, amnesia, or cognitive impairment. Dementia involves loss of memory along with deficits in one or more other area of cognition (i.e., word-finding, verbal expression, comprehension, calculations, attention, judgment, reasoning). It also includes functional loss. To demonstrate this requires a history in which there is report of inability to do something that the individual used to be able to do (functional loss) and a mental status examination that demonstrates loss of more than just memory. [Segal-Gidan F: Dementia, in Moser RL (ed): *Primary Care for Physician Assistants*. New York, McGraw-Hill, 1998, chap 11–5.]

10-5. **The correct answer is B.** There are a number of valid mental status tests that can easily be learned, mastered, and incorporated into routine examinations by any provider. These provide a good means of screening for dementia, particularly among an aging population. The tests, however, are not diagnostic and once deficits can be demonstrated further evaluation is warranted. Individuals with early dementia often fail to report symptoms and family or others may not notice or minimize the early signs of a dementing illness. [Segal-Gidan F: Dementia, in Moser RL (ed): *Primary Care for Physician Assistants*. New York, McGraw-Hill, 1998, chap 11–5.]

10-6. **The correct answer is B.** Hyper- and hypothyroid often present subtly in the elderly. Individuals with dementia may have underlying thyroid disease that is either causative or a contributing factor. Testing for HIV in the presence of dementia is recommended only when there is the presence of risk factors for HIV disease. Urine drug toxicity screening is not routinely performed in the evaluation of dementia or delirium, but may be warranted if drug abuse (legal or illegal) is suspected. ApoE lipoprotein is a genetic test for a marker that has been shown to be related to the development of Alzheimer's disease. It is currently widely available and should be considered in families with a high incidence of dementia, especially Alzheimer's disease, but is not routinely recommended. [Segal-Gidan F: Dementia, in Moser RL (ed): *Primary Care for Physician Assistants*. New York, McGraw-Hill, 1998, chap 11–5.]

10-7.   The correct answer is A.   Normal-pressure hydrocephalus by definition involves the triad of dementia, urinary incontinence, and gait instability. There may be a rapidly progressing dementia, but not an acute confusional state (delirium). In NPH, there is no nausea, vomiting, or other signs of increased intracranial pressure. If these three symptoms are present, especially in the presence of a rapidly progressing dementia, then a CT or MRI scan should be obtained to confirm the presence of ventricular enlargement without sulci prominence and a neurosurgical referral made. Muscle incoordination and swallowing problems, in the presence of a dementia, suggest amyotrophic lateral sclerosis (ALS) or some other neurodegenerative disorder. [Segal-Gidan F: Dementia, in Moser RL (ed): *Primary Care for Physician Assistants.* New York, McGraw-Hill, 1998, chap 11–5.]

10-8.   The correct answer is B.   Acute confusion is often precipitated by a change in medication, most likely an antipsychotic or benzodiazepine. Flurazepam (Dalmane) is a very long-acting (half-life of 72 h) benzodiazepine that is marketed for sleep disturbances. In the elderly, the drug's half-life is increased. With only a few dosages, the drug concentration can build up and cause an acute confusional state. Synthroid is used to treat hypothyroid disease, which in severe cases can present with confusion. Nifedipine is a calcium channel blocker used to treat hypertension and coronary artery disease and has no effect on cognition. Ranitidine is an H_2 blocker used in the treatment of duodenal ulcers and has no effect on cognition. [Segal-Gidan F: Dementia, in Moser RL (ed): *Primary Care for Physician Assistants.* New York, McGraw-Hill, 1998, chap 11–5.]

10-9.   The correct answer is B.   The risk of developing Alzheimer's disease (AD) increases exponentially with age. A number of genetic markers have been located in recent years that are related to the development of AD, but these still account for only a small proportion of all cases. Females are at twice the risk of developing AD, but this still is a smaller risk than advancing age. Aluminum exposure has not been demonstrated to be a significant risk factor in the development of AD. [Segal-Gidan F: Alzheimer's disease, in Moser RL (ed): *Primary Care for Physician Assistants.* New York, McGraw-Hill, 1998, chap 11–4.]

10-10.   The correct answer is C.   The NINCDS-ADRDA in 1984 established the criteria for the diagnosis of Alzheimer's disease. There must be both a clinical diagnosis of dementia consistent with criteria for probable Alzheimer's disease and histopathologic evidence from an autopsy (or biopsy) of the brain that demonstrates tangles and plaques. A clinical diagnosis of dementia without any other known etiology is consistent with a diagnosis of probable AD, not definitive AD. A family history of AD or brain scans in the presence of a dementia are supportive of a diagnosis of probable AD, but not definitive AD. [Segal-Gidan F: Alzheimer's disease, in Moser RL (ed): *Primary Care for Physician Assistants.* New York, McGraw-Hill, 1998, chap 11–4.]

10-11.   The correct answer is D.   There is currently no definitive test for a clinical diagnosis of AD. A brain image, whether CT, MRI, PET, or SPECT, may show patterns consistent with those seen in Alzheimer's disease, but such tests are not diagnostic. The patterns seen on brain images of patients with AD overlap with patterns in other dementias. Genetic testing for apo E only demonstrates a risk for the development of AD and is not diagnostic. [Segal-Gidan F: Alzheimer's disease, in Moser RL (ed): *Primary Care for Physician Assistants.* New York, McGraw-Hill, 1998, chap 11–4.]

10-12.   The correct answer is B.   The presence of new seizures in an individual with dementia, especially in the early stages of the dementia, is inconsistent with a diagnosis of probable AD and should lead the clinician to investigate other, especially intracranial, causes for the dementing process. If no other cause for the dementia can be found in an individual with new-onset seizures and a progressive dementia, then the diagnosis would be possible AD. In probable Alzheimer's disease the brain scan may be normal and the electroencephalogram may show generalized slowing or other abnormalities. The presence of hypertension in an individual with dementia increases the possibility that the underlying etiology is vascular disease, but the presence of hypertension does not exclude a diagnosis of probable AD. [Segal-Gidan F: Alzheimer's disease, in Moser RL (ed): *Primary Care for Physician Assistants*. New York, McGraw-Hill, 1998, chap 11–4.]

10-13.   The correct answer is C.   Tacrine (Cognex) is the only drug currently approved by the FDA for the treatment of Alzheimer's disease. It has been shown to slow down the rate of decline in 15 to 20 percent of individuals in the early stages of probable Alzheimer's disease. The drug can be prescribed by any medical provider licensed to prescribe and, in fact, is more commonly prescribed by primary care providers than neurologists or other specialists. There are no reports of problems taking the medication in the presence of other medications, yet experience has been limited. The drug is hepatotoxic and requires frequent monitoring of liver enzymes during the first several months while dosing is gradually increased. If hepatotoxicity becomes evident by elevated ALT (2 × upper limit of normal), the drug should be stopped. After liver enzymes have returned to normal the drug can be successfully reintroduced with reduced probability of repeat hepatotoxicity. [Segal-Gidan F: Alzheimer's disease, in Moser RL (ed): *Primary Care for Physician Assistants*. New York, McGraw-Hill, 1998, chap 11–4.]

10-14.   The correct answer is B.   In Alzheimer's disease, memory loss is prominent, usually involving recent memory early in the course of the disease and to a greater extent than remote memory. A hallmark of Alzheimer's disease is early deterioration of language, particularly paraphasic errors and expressive aphasias. Poor judgment occurs in Alzheimer's disease, but not usually in the absence of other cognitive deficits, especially memory. Visual problems are not specifically associated with Alzheimer's disease. [Segal-Gidan F: Alzheimer's disease, in Moser RL (ed): *Primary Care for Physician Assistants*. New York, McGraw-Hill, 1998, chap 11–4.]

10-15.   The correct answer is A.   The most common idiopathic localization-related seizure disorder is benign childhood epilepsy with centrotemporal spikes. It is also referred to as benign rolandic epilepsy. It begins between the ages of 3 and 13 years. It manifests as simple partial seizures with sensorimotor symptoms that predominantly affect parts of the face, such as the mouth. [Mosier WA: Seizure disorders (epilepsy), in Moser RL (ed): *Primary Care for Physician Assistants*. New York, McGraw-Hill, 1998, chap 11–1.]

10-16.   The correct answer is A.   The most familiar expression of nonconvulsive seizures is absence seizures. These seizures are sometimes referred to as petit mal seizures. These seizures usually begin in early childhood and thus are sometimes referred to as childhood absence epilepsy (pyknolepsy), juvenile absence epilepsy, or juvenile myoclonic epilepsy. [Mosier WA: Seizure disorders (epilepsy), in Moser RL (ed): *Primary Care for Physician Assistants*. New York, McGraw-Hill, 1998, chap 11–1.]

10-17.   The correct answer is D.   Status epilepticus refers to a seizure that lasts longer than 30 min or a series of seizures with no recovery of full consciousness between attacks. Both generalized and localization-related seizures may progress to status epilepticus. The most common causes of status epilepticus include withdrawal of antiepileptic drugs, sedative-hypnotic drugs, alcohol, high fever, metabolic disorders, and cerebral lesions. [Mosier WA: Seizure disorders (epilepsy), in Moser RL (ed): *Primary Care for Physician Assistants*. New York, McGraw-Hill, 1998, chap 11–1.]

10-18.   The correct answer is E.   Multiple sclerosis is the most commonly occurring demyelinating disease of the CNS. There are approximately 250,000 diagnosed cases in the United States alone. However, some patients may be asymptomatic most or all of their lives. The actual rate is probably higher. This assertion is based on autopsy studies that indicate 20 percent of MS cases are undiagnosed until after death. [Mosier WA: Multiple sclerosis, in Moser RL (ed): *Primary Care for Physician Assistants*. New York, McGraw-Hill, 1998, chap 11–2.]

10-19. **The correct answer is A.** Physical examination findings in a patient with multiple sclerosis may be very different from what the patient perceives to be their major problem. The more common neurologic findings on physical examination of patients with MS involve edema of the optic nerve visualized on funduscopic examination, nystagmus, limb coordination difficulties, abnormal speech patterns, and overactive tendon reflexes. [Mosier WA: Multiple sclerosis, in Moser RL (ed): *Primary Care for Physician Assistants*. New York, McGraw-Hill, 1998, chap 11–2.]

10-20. **The correct answer is C.** Multiple sclerosis is typically a disease of early adulthood. It rarely occurs prior to age 15 or after age 40. The frequency of flare-ups is greatest within the first few years of diagnosis. The first attack, however, may be so mild that it escapes medical attention and may not be followed by a second attack for 10 to 20 years. During typical episodes, symptoms worsen over a period of a few days to a few weeks and then remit. Recovery may occur over a period of weeks or extend over several months. [Mosier WA: Multiple sclerosis, in Moser RL (ed): *Primary Care for Physician Assistants*. New York, McGraw-Hill, 1998, chap 11–2.]

10-21. **The correct answer is A.** Multiple sclerosis is a demyelinating disease of the central nervous system. It attacks the fatty myelin coating of the nerve fibers causing scarring referred to as sclerosis. These plaques of demyelination may occur at multiple sites throughout the brain and spinal cord. [Mosier WA: Multiple sclerosis, in Moser RL (ed): *Primary Care for Physician Assistants*. New York, McGraw-Hill, 1998, chap 11–2.]

10-22. **The correct answer is A.** Diagnosing MS is not easy. There are no diagnostic tests, per se, that unequivocally confirm the disease. In fact, for many patients the diagnosis is reached only after many years of uncertainty and misdiagnosis. How long until a person receives an accurate diagnosis often depends upon the frequency and severity of the symptoms. Special studies can only lend support to a diagnosis that must be made from clinical findings. [Mosier WA: Multiple sclerosis, in Moser RL (ed): *Primary Care for Physician Assistants*. New York, McGraw-Hill, 1998, chap 11–2.]

10-23. **The correct answer is D.** These four features may present in any combination in the patient with Parkinson's disease. To determine the disorder based on one symptom or to diagnose early in the course is very difficult. If Parkinson's disease is suspected, clinical evaluation should also include Meyerson's sign, fixed facial expression, and mild blepharoclonus.[Paterson KB: Parkinson's disease, in Moser RL (ed): *Primary Care for Physician Assistants*. New York, McGraw-Hill, 1998, chap 11–7.]

10-24. **The correct answer is B.** The Lewy body is found in degenerating neurons in most cases of Parkinson's disease. Symptoms such as tremor and postural instability are characteristic of the disorder but may not always be present. If located at all, changes in the globus pallidus are less likely to occur. [Paterson KB: Parkinson's disease, in Moser RL (ed): *Primary Care for Physician Assistants*. New York, McGraw-Hill, 1998, chap 11–7.]

10-25. **The correct answer is E.** Because of the unknown etiology of Parkinson's disease, many excellent drugs are used to treat the disorder symptomatically. Carbidopa-levodopa combinations help to restore dopaminergic function lost in the degeneration of the disease. Beta blockers and anticholinergics help control the progress of the disease as well as suppress symptoms. These three groups form the basis of medication treatment for Parkinson's disease patients. [Paterson KB: Parkinson's disease, in Moser RL (ed): *Primary Care for Physician Assistants*. New York, McGraw-Hill, 1998, chap 11–7.]

10-26. **The correct answer is D.**   Myasthenia gravis is considered a neuromuscular auto-immune disease. Circulating antibodies destroy acetylcholine receptor sites located on the postganglionic membrane of the neuromuscular junction. Plasmapheresis effectively eliminates circulating antibodies found in 80 percent of myasthenic patients and temporarily alleviates symptoms. [Stephanoff CC: Myasthenia gravis, in Moser RL (ed): *Primary Care for Physician Assistants*. New York, McGraw-Hill, 1998, chap 11–6.]

10-27. **The correct answer is A.**   Myasthenia gravis is a disease of the myoneural junction. Chemical transfer of action potentials from the presynaptic to postsynaptic membrane is severely decreased. As a result, insufficient sarcolemma recruitment yields loss of muscular strength and endurance. Treatment with an anticholinesterase agent temporarily reverses these symptoms. [Stephanoff CC: Myasthenia gravis, in Moser RL (ed): *Primary Care for Physician Assistants*. New York, McGraw-Hill, 1998, chap 11–6.]

10-28. **The correct answer is D.**   Circulating acetylcholine receptors antibodies (AChR-ab) are responsible for the destruction of acetylcholine receptors. Approximately 80 percent of myasthenic patients have detectable serum AChR-ab. Plasmapheresis is a treatment modality that removes antibodies from the patient's blood and temporarily alleviates symptoms. [Stephanoff CC: Myasthenia gravis, in Moser RL (ed): *Primary Care for Physician Assistants*. New York, McGraw-Hill, 1998, chap 11–6.]

10-29. **The correct answer is B.**   The presumed location of the nausea reaction is the chemoreceptor trigger zone in the midbrain area. CN X mediates the sensation. Since the vagus enervates a multitude of areas, many of which deal with our vital signs and restorative systems (digestive), it is not surprising that many disease processes present with nausea and progress to vomiting. [Heinly AP: Nausea and vomiting, in Moser RL (ed): *Primary Care for Physician Assistants*. New York, McGraw-Hill, 1998, chap 6–19.]

SECTION 11
OBSTETRICS/GYNECOLOGY

11. OBSTETRICS/GYNECOLOGY

QUESTIONS

DIRECTIONS: Each question below contains suggested responses. Choose the **one best** response to each question.

11-1. A 22-year-old aerobic instructor complains of burning on urination and intense itching in the vaginal area for the past 2 days. A thick whitish discharge was noted on the labia. The probable diagnosis is

(A) trichomoniasis
(B) vulvovaginal candidiasis
(C) bacterial vaginosis
(D) gonococcal urethritis

11-2. A patient presents with severe vulvar irritation and thick white vaginal discharge. Potassium hydroxide (KOH) preparation is positive for budding yeast and pseudohyphae. The preferred treatment is

(A) metronidazole 2 g PO in a single dose
(B) miconazole 2% cream 5 g intravaginally × 7 days
(C) clotrimazole 500 mg vaginal tablet in a single application
(D) fluconazole 100 mg PO bid × 7 days

11-3. All of the following symptoms are usually associated with vulvovaginal candidiasis EXCEPT

(A) dyspareunia
(B) vulvar burning
(C) external dysuria
(D) malodorous discharge

11-4. All of the following are signs and symptoms that may be associated with vaginal trichomoniasis EXCEPT

(A) yellow-green vaginal discharge
(B) vulvar irritation
(C) strawberry cervix
(D) clumped white vaginal discharge

11-5. The diagnosis of vaginal trichomoniasis is BEST made by

(A) observing a greenish-yellow frothy vaginal discharge
(B) history of unprotected sexual intercourse and a vaginal discharge
(C) observing motile parasites by microscopy
(D) dipstick for detection of leukocytes

11-6. The treatment of choice for vaginal trichomoniasis is

(A) metronidazole 2 g PO in a single dose
(B) metronidazole 500 mg PO twice daily for 7 days
(C) metronidazole gel 5 g intravaginally for 3 days
(D) clotrimazole 500 mg vaginal tablet in a single application

11-7. The discharge in bacterial vaginosis can be described as

(A) purulent, causing inflammation of the vaginal mucosa
(B) white, noninflammatory, with fishy odor
(C) thick and creamy, causing mild irritation to vaginal wall
(D) greenish-yellow and frothy, with a foul smell

11-8. The treatment of choice for bacterial vaginosis is

(A) metronidazole 500 mg PO twice daily for 7 days
(B) metronidazole 2 g PO in a single dose
(C) clindamycin cream 2% one full applicator (5g) intravaginally HS for 7 days
(D) clindamycin 300 mg PO twice daily for 7 days

11-9. Which of the following sexually transmitted diseases has the HIGHEST incidence of transmission after a sexual assault?

(A) chlamydia
(B) gonorrhea
(C) herpes simplex virus
(D) human immunodeficiency virus
(E) trichomonas vaginalis

11-10. All of the following medications should be offered as prophylaxis after a sexual assault EXCEPT

(A) ceftriaxone
(B) doxycycline
(C) metronidazole
(D) Ovral (morning-after pill)
(E) terconazole

11-11. Initial diagnostic tests recommended by the CDC for sexually transmitted diseases after a sexual assault include all the following EXCEPT

(A) chlamydia culture
(B) gonorrhea culture
(C) herpes simplex virus serology
(D) wet prep for bacterial vaginosis
(E) wet prep for trichomonas vaginalis

11-12. Polycystic ovary syndrome is characterized by

(A) hyperandrogenism and chronic anovulation
(B) hypothyroidism and amenorrhea
(C) obesity and infertility
(D) dyslipidemia and dysfunctional uterine bleeding
(E) insulin resistance and oligomenorrhea

11-13. The cause of polycystic ovary syndrome is

(A) excess prolactin
(B) hypothyroidism
(C) insulin resistance
(D) overdose of exogenous estrogen
(E) unknown

11-14. The "gold standard" for diagnosing polycystic ovary syndrome is

(A) pelvic CT
(B) pelvic sonogram
(C) serum LH, FSH, and TSH
(D) serum testosterone
(E) serum androstenedione

11-15. The cause of premenstrual syndrome (PMS) is

(A) estrogen/progesterone imbalance
(B) vitamin B_6 deficiency
(C) serotonin deficiency
(D) psychiatric
(E) unknown

11-16. A diagnosis of PMS is made when

(A) elevated estrogen and low progesterone serum levels are demonstrated, especially when drawn on day 21 of the menstrual cycle
(B) serum B_6 is below normal
(C) Prozac used presumptively treats the symptoms successfully
(D) 3 months of daily symptom charting reveals cyclic symptoms starting at ovulation and abating with menses
(E) all criteria as described in the DSM-IV are met

11-17. A 49-year-old female patient presents with a chief complaint of cyclic irritability, depression, and fatigue. Occasionally she has night sweats, but these are barely even noticeable. A complete physical exam with lab last month was completely normal. In considering a diagnosis of PMS, what is the MOST important initial question to ask this patient?

(A) "Are you under psychiatric care?"
(B) "Are you having monthly periods?"
(C) "Do you have a thyroid condition?"
(D) "Have you ever been treated for vitamin deficiency?"
(E) "What medications are you taking?"

11-18. A 37-year-old female patient has carried out your instructions to keep a daily symptom chart for PMS. After 4 months, her charting shows the classic pattern of symptomatology and the diagnosis of PMS is made. Because she has had severe affective symptoms that have been largely unresponsive to diet and exercise changes, she requests further treatments. Your next course of action would be

(A) refer her to a psychiatrist
(B) offer her a trial course of selective serotonin reuptake inhibitors (SSRIs)
(C) suggest high doses of Vitamin B complex daily
(D) prescribe micronized progesterone 300 mg qid
(E) prescribe alprazolam 0.25 mg once daily, day 18 until menses

11-19. One of your patients with PMS has had a very successful treatment regimen that includes a low-sugar, low-salt, and no-caffeine diet; regular jogging; and a complete vitamin/mineral supplementation program. Lately she is noticing that premenstrual bloating is becoming a bit more prominent, but worse, she is quite fatigued and labile 1 to 2 days before her period. She prefers not to use medications, and would like recommendations about additional nondrug measures. You suggest

(A) attending a local support group for women with PMS
(B) discontinuing exercise, as it accentuates the bloating and fatigue
(C) using moderate amounts of caffeine as a diuretic and to fight fatigue
(D) doubling her vitamin dosages
(E) abandoning this regimen because it's not working

11-20. An 18-year-old grav 0/para 0 patient has been successfully treated for *Neisseria gonorrhoeae* salpingitis and asks about her risk of infertility. Based on this single infection her chances of infertility are approximately

(A) <1 percent
(B) 3 to 5 percent
(C) 10 to 15 percent
(D) 20 to 25 percent
(E) 30 to 35 percent

11-21. On her first prenatal visit, a 26-year-old primigravida patient at 14 weeks gestation has a positive culture for gonorrhea. The drug of choice for the treatment of gonorrhea in this patient would be

(A) ciprofloxacin
(B) ceftriaxone
(C) doxycycline
(D) ampicillin
(E) Bicillin CR

11-22. The MOST common presenting symptom in women with gonorrhea is a(n)

(A) vaginal discharge
(B) genital ulcer
(C) perineal pruritus
(D) asymptomatic patient

11-23. On her first prenatal visit, a 24-year-old primigravida patient at 12 weeks gestation has a positive culture result for chlamydia. The drug of choice for the treatment of chlamydia in this patient would be

(A) doxycycline
(B) erythromycin base
(C) penicillin
(D) ceftriaxone
(E) vancomycin

11-24. Risk factors associated with the acquisition of pelvic inflammatory disease (PID) include all the following EXCEPT

(A) age >25 years old
(B) presence of an IUD
(C) recent invasive gynecologic procedure
(D) smoking
(E) vaginal douching

11-25. Which of the following laboratory tests can be ordered initially to help make the diagnosis in a patient with suspected PID?

(A) CBC
(B) culdocentesis
(C) endometrial biopsy
(D) laparoscopy
(E) pap smear

11-26. The initiation of treatment for presumed PID is based on

(A) cervical Gram stain results
(B) clinical suspicion
(C) rebound tenderness
(D) serology results
(E) white blood cell count

11-27. Toxic shock syndrome is caused by a toxin produced by which microorganism?

(A) *C. difficile*
(B) *E. coli*
(C) *S. aureus*
(D) *S. pyogenes*
(E) *S. viridans*

11-28. What percentages of women who develop toxic shock syndrome have recurrences with subsequent menses?

(A) 10 percent
(B) 20 percent
(C) 30 percent
(D) 40 percent
(E) 50 percent

11-29. Which of the following symptoms of menopause is MOST prevalent?

(A) vaginal dryness
(B) decreased libido
(C) hot flashes
(D) nervousness
(E) mood swings

11-30. The MOST useful biochemical marker of menopause is

(A) an elevated TSH
(B) increased serum testosterone
(C) elevated estradiol level
(D) increased FSH
(E) low serum albumin

11-31. Adding a progestin in a cyclic or continuous fashion to the hormone replacement therapy regimen

(A) improves HDL levels
(B) prevents endometrial hyperplasia
(C) reduces the risk of pregnancy
(D) augments the action of estrogen
(E) eliminates the risk of gallbladder disease

11-32. The combined continuous regimen of hormone replacement therapy in menopause is popular because

(A) many women will completely stop bleeding after 6 months
(B) after 6 months therapy can be stopped altogether
(C) there are no bothersome side effects
(D) it is the most cost-effective form of therapy
(E) there is significant improvement in libido

11-33. Which is MOST effective in preventing bone loss in a woman with premature menopause?

(A) high calcium intake
(B) increased vitamin D
(C) estrogen
(D) bisphosphonate
(E) calcitonin

11-34. Which of the following women needs a higher starting dose of estrogen when initiating therapy?

(A) a 52-year-old woman with 6 to 10 hot flashes per day
(B) a 38-year-old smoker who has had a recent hysterectomy
(C) a 49-year-old with no hot flashes; 8 months of amenorrhea
(D) a 50-year-old woman who has been physically inactive before menopause
(E) a 51-year-old woman with a history of breast cancer

11-35. A new mother, immediately postpartum, presents in your office with gradual onset, bilateral breast pain. Other than being tired, she feels well, but is concerned about her breast discomfort. A physical examination reveals an afebrile patient with hard breasts and nipples that are tender to palpation. Your diagnosis is

(A) plugged breast duct
(B) mastitis
(C) engorgement
(D) inflammatory breast cancer
(E) tuberculosis, disseminated

11-36. Three months later, this now-experienced nursing mother (see question 11-35) presents with one-sided breast soreness. The patient is very concerned about a new breast lump that is just slightly red and warm. Your patient has been feeling quite well. In fact, she has started a new exercise program and frequently takes the baby for long walks, using a baby carrier. Your diagnosis now is

(A) plugged breast duct
(B) mastitis
(C) engorgement
(D) inflammatory breast cancer
(E) tuberculosis, disseminated

11-37. The MOST important supportive measure to take in treating mastitis is

(A) early weaning to let the breast heal
(B) wearing a nursing bra at all times for added support
(C) applying ice locally to numb breast pain
(D) nursing frequently and emptying the breast completely
(E) taking acetaminophen to facilitate nursing despite breast pain

11-38. Which of the following is the LEAST common cause of uterine prolapse?

(A) rectocele
(B) cystocele
(C) enterocele
(D) urethrocele
(E) uterocele

11-39. Which of the following is the MOST common cause of a herniation of the posterior vaginal wall?

(A) rectocele
(B) cystocele
(C) enterocele
(D) urethrocele
(E) hydrocele

11-40. All of the following are absolute contraindications to combined oral contraceptive use. All are also absolute contraindications to use of progestin-only contraceptives EXCEPT

(A) active thromboembolic disorder
(B) hypertension
(C) pregnancy
(D) undiagnosed abnormal genital bleeding
(E) breast cancer

11-41. Your patient is a 35-year-old mother of three in a mutually monogamous relationship who has recently been found to have elevated liver function tests. You advise her to avoid pregnancy while undergoing evaluation to determine the etiology of her hepatic dysfunction. She asks you for advice on the most effective contraceptive method she can safely use. Your answer is

(A) condoms alone
(B) Depo-Provera
(C) diaphragm
(D) IUD
(E) combined oral contraceptives

11-42. All of the following statements regarding breast cysts are TRUE EXCEPT

(A) They occur commonly in adolescent women.
(B) They occur most commonly in postmenopausal women.
(C) They frequently resolve with needle aspiration.
(D) Clear aspirate from cysts does not routinely require cytologic examination.
(E) Their presence does not raise a higher than average suspicion of breast cancer.

11-43. Five clinical situations are presented. Mammography is contraindicated in two of them, and may be misleading in two others. In which clinical situation presented below is mammography of great benefit?

(A) A 40-year-old woman discovered a hard, fixed mass that yielded no tissue on needle biopsy. Mammograms have been ordered prior to excisional biopsy to rule out occult cancer.

(B) A 32-year-old woman has been found to have a persistent, firm, mobile mass in her left breast. Her sister had breast cancer at age 42. She requests a mammogram so that she does not have to worry that her mass might be cancer.

(C) A 19-year-old woman presents with a soft mass that is most palpable before her period, and nearly resolves the week following her menses. Her mother, whose sister has recently been diagnosed with breast cancer, has encouraged her to have a mammogram to rule out cancer.

(D) A 38-year-old woman presents for a scheduled screening mammogram. She missed her period the week before but had not really considered the possibility that she might be pregnant. She took the day off from work, has waited several weeks for this appointment, and sees no harm in having the mammogram performed.

(E) A 45-year-old woman with a long history of multiple breast cysts has a lump that feels different to her than her usual cysts. Her clinician orders a mammogram so she will not need an unnecessary biopsy referral.

11-44. The MOST common symptom of a prolactinoma in women is

(A) visual field defect
(B) headache
(C) galactorrhea
(D) facial numbness
(E) amenorrhea

11-45. Transient hypothyroidism following pregnancy is

(A) rare
(B) best treated with NSAIDs
(C) an indication for permanent levothyroxine replacement
(D) an indication for levothyroxine replacement
(E) not likely to recur

11. OBSTETRICS/GYNECOLOGY

ANSWERS

11-1. The correct answer is B. The classic symptoms for vulvovaginal candidiasis include itching and whitish discharge. The discharge of trichomonas is usually greenish yellow. Bacterial vaginosis does not cause an inflammatory response nor itching or burning. Gonococcal urethritis is not a cause of vaginal pruritus, and the discharge is usually purulent. [Valentine P: Vulvovaginal candidiasis, in Moser RL (ed): *Primary Care for Physician Assistants*. New York, McGraw-Hill, 1998, chap 12–2.]

11-2. The correct answer is B. All agents are antifungal, but miconazole is the preferred answer based on 7-day therapy for an acute case of vulvovaginal candidiasis. Single-dose therapy with clotrimazole is reserved for uncomplicated mild to moderate vulvovaginal candidiasis. Fluconazole is thought to prevent recurrence of vulvovaginal candidiasis, and the 100 mg is offered weekly. Metronidazole is used to treat trichomonas and bacterial vaginosis. [Valentine P: Vulvovaginal candidiasis, in Moser RL (ed): *Primary Care for Physician Assistants*. New York, McGraw-Hill, 1998, chap 12–2.]

11-3. The correct answer is D. Malodorous discharge is rarely associated with vulvovaginal candidiasis. Choices A, B, and C are frequent complaints in patients with vulvovaginal candidiasis. [Valentine P: Vulvovaginal candidiasis, in Moser RL (ed): *Primary Care for Physician Assistants*. New York, McGraw-Hill, 1998, chap 12–2.]

11-4. The correct answer is D. Clumped white discharge is usually associated with vaginal yeast infection. Yellow-green discharge and vulvar irritation are classically seen in trichomoniasis. Strawberry cervix is observed in 1 to 2 percent of the cases during speculum examination, but observed 50 percent of the time by colposcopy when *Trichomonas* is present. [Valentine P: Trichomoniasis, in Moser RL (ed): *Primary Care for Physician Assistants*. New York, McGraw-Hill, 1998, chap 12–11.]

11-5. The correct answer is C. Observation of motile parasites confirms the diagnosis. History and symptoms alone do not establish the diagnosis. Frothy discharge may be noted in bacterial vaginosis as well, and dipstick detection of leukocytes is useful in determining the presence of cystitis. [Valentine P: Trichomoniasis, in Moser RL (ed): *Primary Care for Physician Assistants*. New York, McGraw-Hill, 1998, chap 12–11.]

11-6. The correct answer is A. Metronidazole for 7 days is an alternative treatment, and the gel has not been studied for treatment of trichomoniasis. Clotrimazole is an antifungal agent. [Valentine P: Trichomoniasis, in Moser RL (ed): *Primary Care for Physician Assistants*. New York, McGraw-Hill, 1998, chap 12–11.]

11-7. The correct answer is B. The discharge in bacterial vaginosis can occasionally be yellow, but is most often white or gray. Rarely would one note inflammation of the mucosa, unless a coexisting condition is present, e.g., trichomonas. C is most often associated with yeast infection, and D is most often seen in trichomoniasis. [Valentine P: Bacterial vaginosis, in Moser RL (ed): *Primary Care for Physician Assistants*. New York, McGraw-Hill, 1998, chap 12–3.]

11-8. **The correct answer is A.** All of the other choices are alternative therapies for treating bacterial vaginosis. [Valentine P: Bacterial vaginosis, in Moser RL (ed): *Primary Care for Physician Assistants*. New York, McGraw-Hill, 1998, chap 12–3.]

11-9. **The correct answer is B.** The risk of contracting an STD is associated with the degree of sexual contact and the number of assailants. Gonorrhea has been isolated in up to 13 percent of all reported sexual assaults. [Covino JM: Sexual assault, in Moser RL (ed): *Primary Care for Physician Assistants*. New York, McGraw-Hill, 1998, chap 12–10.]

11-10. **The correct answer is E.** Although not all experts agree, most patients do benefit from prophylaxis. The regimen recommended by the Centers for Disease Control includes ceftriaxone 125 mg IM + metronidazole 2g PO stat dose + doxycycline 100 mg bid × 7 days. The "morning after" contraceptive therapy should be offered to any childbearing woman who was raped less than 72 h previous. Terconazole is used for vaginal yeast infections and is not part of the prophylaxis regimen. [Covino JM: Sexual assault, in Moser RL (ed): *Primary Care for Physician Assistants*. New York, McGraw-Hill, 1998, chap 12–10.]

11-11. **The correct answer is C.** The CDC recommends the following initial diagnostic tests for STDs after a sexual assault: gonorrhea and chlamydia cultures, wet mount for bacterial vaginosis and *Trichomonas*, and a blood sample to be saved for subsequent analysis. [Covino JM: Sexual assault, in Moser RL (ed): *Primary Care for Physician Assistants*. New York, McGraw-Hill, 1998, chap 12–10.]

11-12. **The correct answer is A.** Hyperandrogenism may manifest clinically as hirsutism, acne, and alopecia; chronic anovulation may cause a variety of menstrual irregularities including amenorrhea, oligomenorrhea, and infertility. While dyslipidemia and insulin resistance are associated with polycystic ovary, not everyone with polycystic ovary syndrome (PCOS) has these conditions. Although it may complicate an individual case, hypothyroidism is an entity distinct from PCOS. Obesity occurs in about half of women with polycystic ovary syndrome. [Gallagher DM: Polycystic ovary syndrome, in Moser RL (ed): *Primary Care for Physician Assistants*. New York, McGraw-Hill, 1998, chap 12–9.]

11-13. **The correct answer is E.** Historically, the cause of polycystic ovary syndrome was attributed to a disorder of the hypothalamic-pituitary-ovarian pathway, causing hyperandrogenism. More recently, hyperinsulinism has been implicated as a precursor to hyperandrogenism; however, the mechanism of pathogenicity remains unclear. [Gallagher DM: Polycystic ovary syndrome, in Moser RL (ed): *Primary Care for Physician Assistants*. New York, McGraw-Hill, 1998, chap 12–9.]

11-14. **The correct answer is B.** Contemporary ultrasound images are considered quite reliable, as they correlate with histology in better than 90 percent of cases. There is no serum test that clinches the diagnosis of polycystic ovary syndrome (PCOS). Hypersecretion of testosterone, androstenedione, and LH may be seen with PCOS, but normal values do not rule it out. Pelvic CT is not an appropriate diagnostic tool. [Gallagher DM: Polycystic ovary syndrome, in Moser RL (ed): *Primary Care for Physician Assistants*. New York, McGraw-Hill, 1998, chap 12–9.]

11-15. **The correct answer is E.** Although many theories as to etiology have been proposed, none have been proven. The National Institute of Child Health and Human Development is currently conducting a study of the interrelationships of hypothalamic, pituitary, and ovarian function; one of the hoped-for discoveries is the cause of premenstrual syndrome. [Gallagher DM: Premenstrual syndrome, in Moser RL (ed): *Primary Care for Physician Assistants*. New York, McGraw-Hill, 1998, chap 12–4.]

11-16. **The correct answer is D.** At this time, there are no lab, radiologic, or clinical diagnostic tests for the detection of PMS. The diagnosis rests on the documentation of cyclic physical and/or affective symptoms, which occur in the interim between ovulation and menses. [Gallagher DM: Premenstrual syndrome, in Moser RL (ed): *Primary Care for Physician Assistants*. New York, McGraw-Hill, 1998, chap 12–4.]

11-17.   The correct answer is B.   The single most important piece of information about this woman is her menstrual status, because it dictates your workup. If the patient has irregular or no menses, perimenopause is a likely cause of her symptoms. If the patient has monthly cycles, daily symptom charting should be initiated. [Gallagher DM: Premenstrual syndrome, in Moser RL (ed): *Primary Care for Physician Assistants*. New York, McGraw-Hill, 1998, chap 12–4.]

11-18.   The correct answer is B.   Prozac has been shown to improve affective PMS symptoms in 50 percent of women. There is no evidence to support the use of vitamins or progesterone for affective symptoms of PMS. Treatment with alprazolam should be reserved for cases not improved by use of SSRIs. [Gallagher DM: Premenstrual syndrome, in Moser RL (ed): *Primary Care for Physician Assistants*. New York, McGraw-Hill, 1998, chap 12–4.]

11-19.   The correct answer is A.   Since the patient refuses medications, and other nondrug treatments are unproven, the remaining additional suggestion for a woman with affective symptoms would be to seek support. Her current regimen is healthful overall and not contributing to her symptoms, so it should be continued. [Gallagher DM: Premenstrual syndrome, in Moser RL (ed): *Primary Care for Physician Assistants*. New York, McGraw-Hill, 1998, chap 12–4.]

11-20.   The correct answer is C.   About 11 percent of women are infertile after a single episode of pelvic inflammatory disease (PID), 23 percent after two episodes, and over 50 percent after three or more episodes. The increased risk of infertility and ectopic pregnancy is directly related to duration of symptoms before treatment. Nongonococcal infection predisposes more commonly to ectopic pregnancy, and thus carries a worse prognosis for a subsequent viable pregnancy. [Covino JM: Pelvic inflammatory disease, in Moser RL (ed): *Primary Care for Physician Assistants*. New York, McGraw-Hill, 1998, chap 12–8.]

11-21.   The correct answer is B.   Ceftriaxone is the treatment of choice for pregnant patients with gonorrhea. [Hansen M: Gonorrhea, in Moser RL (ed): *Primary Care for Physician Assistants*. New York, McGraw-Hill, 1998, chap 9–13.]

11-22.   The correct answer is A.   A vaginal discharge, often copious, is a common presenting symptom in gonorrhea in females. A genital ulcer is more likely to be herpetic or syphilitic, whereas pruritus is more common with a yeast infection. Although women may be asymptomatic and have gonorrhea, more often this is not the case. [Hansen M: Gonorrhea, in Moser RL (ed): *Primary Care for Physician Assistants*. New York, McGraw-Hill, 1998, chap 9–13.]

11-23.   The correct answer is B.   The usual drug of choice, doxycycline, cannot be used in pregnancy, so erythromycin is the preferred drug. [Hansen M: Chlamydia, in Moser RL (ed): *Primary Care for Physician Assistants*. New York, McGraw-Hill, 1998, chap 9–6.]

11-24.   The correct answer is A.   Certain risk factors have been associated with PID and should be sought while taking a history from any women with lower abdominal pain. PID is more prevalent in the younger population (age <25 years old). [Covino JM: Pelvic inflammatory disease, in Moser RL (ed): *Primary Care for Physician Assistants*. New York, McGraw-Hill, 1998, chap 12–8.]

11-25.   The correct answer is A.   White blood count may be elevated in acute cases of PID. Culdocentesis, endometrial biopsy, and laparoscopy are invasive techniques and are reserved for cases where the diagnosis is imperative but remains uncertain. Pap smear results do not help in diagnosing PID. [Covino JM: Pelvic inflammatory disease, in Moser RL (ed): *Primary Care for Physician Assistants*. New York, McGraw-Hill, 1998, chap 12–8.]

11-26. **The correct answer is B.** Even though the other findings may or may not be present, the initiation of treatment for presumed PID can be based on clinical suspicion. It is not imperative that specific objective findings or laboratory tests be present in order to treat a patient. [Covino JM: Pelvic inflammatory disease, in Moser RL (ed): *Primary Care for Physician Assistants.* New York, McGraw-Hill, 1998, chap 12–8.]

11-27. **The correct answer is C.** The cause of toxic shock syndrome (TSS) is preformed toxins produced by *S. aureus,* so that colonization or infection by this microorganism must occur. [Covino JM: Toxic shock syndrome, in Moser RL (ed): *Primary Care for Physician Assistants.* New York, McGraw-Hill, 1998, chap 9–24.]

11-28. **The correct answer is C.** Approximately 30 percent of women who develop TSS have recurrences. The greatest risk for recurrence is during the first three menstrual periods following treatment, and the recurrent episode may be less or more severe than the initial one. The incidence is reduced to less than 5 percent if antistaphylococcal antibiotic therapy is given during therapy of the initial occurrence. [Covino JM: Toxic shock syndrome, in Moser RL (ed): *Primary Care for Physician Assistants.* New York, McGraw-Hill, 1998, chap 9–24.]

11-29. **The correct answer is C.** All of the symptoms listed can occur in menopause. However, hot flashes are the most prevalent. Close to 75 percent of women will experience hot flashes at some time during menopause. [Hess L: Menopause, in Moser RL (ed): *Primary Care for Physician Assistants.* New York, McGraw-Hill, 1998, chap 12–17.]

11-30. **The correct answer is D.** An increased FSH is the most sensitive biochemical marker of menopause. An FSH level of greater than 30 mIU/mL defines menopause. Estradiol levels decrease in menopause. The TSH and serum albumin do not change in menopause. The testosterone levels of women tend to decrease slightly after menopause. [Hess L: Menopause, in Moser RL (ed): *Primary Care for Physician Assistants.* New York, McGraw-Hill, 1998, chap 12–17.]

11-31. **The correct answer is B.** It has been documented by numerous studies that adding progestin in a cyclic or continuous fashion to a woman's hormone replacement regimen eliminates the risk of endometrial cancer by preventing endometrial hyperplasia. Women who are taking unopposed estrogens have an endometrial cancer risk 10 times that of women not taking estrogen. [Hess L: Menopause, in Moser RL (ed): *Primary Care for Physician Assistants.* New York, McGraw-Hill, 1998, chap 12–17.]

11-32. **The correct answer is A.** The greatest benefit of the combined continuous therapy (Premarin and Provera taken daily) is that many women (70 percent) will stop bleeding altogether after 6 to 9 months. This is something that most women would like, since monthly or intermittent bleeding is often seen as a bother after menopause. This has become the most popular regimen in the past 5 years. [Hess L: Menopause, in Moser RL (ed): *Primary Care for Physician Assistants.* New York, McGraw-Hill, 1998, chap 12–17.]

11-33. **The correct answer is C.** The cause of bone density loss in premature menopause is low estrogen. Treatment with estrogen replacement is not only the most physiologic therapy, but is the one with the best documented efficacy and safety. Each of the other choices are also effective. [Hess L: Menopause, in Moser RL (ed): *Primary Care for Physician Assistants.* New York, McGraw-Hill, 1998, chap 12–17.]

11-34. **The correct answer is B.** Both smoking and the fact that this woman is having a sudden menopause (hysterectomy) may mean that her requirement for estrogen replacement will be higher. It is felt that thin women, women who smoke more than 15 cigarettes per day, women who have recently had a hysterectomy, and women with increased metabolism will require increased doses of estrogen to alleviate symptoms. [Hess L: Menopause, in Moser RL (ed): *Primary Care for Physician Assistants.* New York, McGraw-Hill, 1998, chap 12–17.]

11-35.   **The correct answer is C.**   Engorgement is the distention of the breast with milk, and is a signal to nurse, not a pathologic state. Breast tenderness and hardness is relieved by emptying the breast completely. [Gallagher DM: Mastitis, in Moser RL (ed): *Primary Care for Physician Assistants.* New York, McGraw-Hill, 1998, chap 12–7.]

11-36.   **The correct answer is A.**   Plugged ducts typically present as a unilateral breast lump with minor localized erythema and heat. Plugged ducts are caused by feedings that are too short and by obstruction of the duct (in this case, by the baby carrier). [Gallagher DM: Mastitis, in Moser RL (ed): *Primary Care for Physician Assistants.* New York, McGraw-Hill, 1998, chap 12–7.]

11-37.   **The correct answer is D.**   Although the impulse may be to provide immediate rest from nursing, weaning during mastitis will stop the breast drainage that is critical to successful treatment. Heat, not ice, should be applied locally. Taking acetaminophen to dull pain is a personal choice for the nursing mother. If a nursing bra provides comfort, it can be worn at all times, but it should be checked for tightness that could interfere with breast drainage. [Gallagher DM: Mastitis, in Moser RL (ed): *Primary Care for Physician Assistants.* New York, McGraw-Hill, 1998, chap 12–7.]

11-38.   **The correct answer is A.**   Of all the types of prolapse, the pure rectocele is the least common. It is usually associated with a cystocele, some degree of uterine descent, and laceration of the perineum. It only occurs when there has been injury to all of the structures that make up the pelvic floor. [Mosier WA: Cystocele and rectocele, in Moser RL (ed): *Primary Care for Physician Assistants.* New York, McGraw-Hill, 1998, chap 12–5.]

11-39.   **The correct answer is A.**   A rectocele is a rectovaginal hernia that results from trauma to the levator muscles and causes a bulging of the anterior rectal wall into the posterior vaginal wall. The rectocele cannot occur without a definite fascial defect associated with a congenital or inherent weakness. [Mosier WA: Cystocele and rectocele, in Moser RL (ed): *Primary Care for Physician Assistants.* New York, McGraw-Hill, 1998, chap 12–5.]

11-40.   **The correct answer is B.**   The difference between combined oral contraceptives and progestin-only methods is estrogen. This question refers to contraindications that are referable to use of estrogen, but not progesterone. Estrogen is implicated as the cause of several important side effects of oral contraceptives, including myocardial infarction, stroke, and hypertension. Progesterone-only methods may be used with caution in the presence of history of all of these illnesses. However, progestin-only methods are absolutely contraindicated in all of the other clinical situations listed in the question. [Genova NJ: Contraception, in Moser RL (ed): *Primary Care for Physician Assistants.* New York, McGraw-Hill, 1998, chap 12–14.]

11-41.   **The correct answer is D.**   Note that the clinician has initiated the topic of contraception in this scenario. The couple may desire a pregnancy, and may be requesting a highly effective method in order to avoid the possibility of a pregnancy that would be dangerous to both the woman and the fetus, especially if abortion is unacceptable. Hormonal contraceptive methods, while very effective, are contraindicated in women with hepatic dysfunction, as they are metabolized in the liver and can exacerbate liver damage. Barrier methods are not as effective as the correct choice, IUD. (Wilson's disease as the cause of the elevated liver function tests would have to be ruled out before insertion of a copper-containing IUD.) Surgical sterilization for either partner could have been included in the choices, but permanent limitation of family size must be decided upon independently by the couple, not recommended by the clinician. [Genova NJ: Contraception, in Moser RL (ed): *Primary Care for Physician Assistants.* New York, McGraw-Hill, 1998, chap 12–14.]

11-42. **The correct answer is B.**   Breast cysts are very common in premenopausal women. Unless they are painful or otherwise bothersome to the woman, their major significance is the need to prove that they do not represent a malignant mass. This may be done by obtaining clear fluid from the cyst by needle biopsy. [Genova NJ: Breast mass, in Moser RL (ed): *Primary Care for Physician Assistants*. New York, McGraw-Hill, 1998, chap 12–12.]

11-43. **The correct answer is A.**   Though the radiation levels used in current mammography techniques are low, they are of most danger in very young and pregnant women. Mammography is contraindicated in scenarios C and D. Scenarios B and E represent "setups" for failure to diagnose breast cancer. Further evaluation in either of these cases CANNOT be avoided by obtaining a normal mammogram. In scenario A, both biopsy and mammography are required, the former for definitive diagnosis of the primary dominant mass, and the latter to detect cancer in either breast, which might not yet be palpable, but which is present in 3 percent of cases. The presence or absence of occult cancer, especially in the contralateral breast, will affect immediate and future treatment decisions. [Genova NJ: Breast mass, in Moser RL (ed): *Primary Care for Physician Assistants*. New York, McGraw-Hill, 1998, chap 12–12.]

11-44. **The correct answer is E.**   Amenorrhea is an early sign of increased prolactin in women, because hyperprolactinemia decreases LH and FSH. Galactorrhea is the second most common associated symptom. The menstrual abnormality usually leads to early diagnosis of prolactinomas as microadenomas in women, so that the macroadenoma symptoms of visual field defect and headache are usually absent. Facial numbness is not a symptom of pituitary tumors. [Evans TC: Anterior pituitary disorders, in Moser RL (ed): *Primary Care for Physician Assistants*. New York, McGraw-Hill, 1998, chap 5–6.]

11-45. **The correct answer is D.**   Postpartum thyroiditis occurs after about 5 percent of pregnancies and may have an initial mild hyperthyroid phase followed by a more prolonged hypothyroid phase, which should be treated with levothyroxine replacement. It is usually a transient dysfunction, however, so replacement therapy should be discontinued after about a year and the TSH followed. This syndrome occurs primarily in patients with underlying autoimmune thyroiditis, so is likely to recur with subsequent pregnancies. [Evans TC: Hypothyroidism, in Moser RL (ed): *Primary Care for Physician Assistants*. New York, McGraw-Hill, 1998, chap 5–3.]

SECTION 12
ONCOLOGY

12. ONCOLOGY

QUESTIONS

DIRECTIONS: Each question below contains suggested responses. Choose the **one best** response to each question.

12-1. Which of the following is the LEADING cause of cancer death in the United States?

- (A) breast cancer
- (B) lung cancer
- (C) colorectal cancer
- (D) prostate cancer
- (E) none of the above

12-2. Which type of lung cancer is exquisitely sensitive to chemotherapy?

- (A) squamous cell carcinoma
- (B) adenocarcinoma
- (C) large cell carcinoma
- (D) small cell carcinoma
- (E) none of the above

12-3. Which of the following groups has an increased incidence of pancreatic cancer?

- (A) Caucasians
- (B) African-Americans
- (C) Hispanics
- (D) males
- (E) females

12-4. The average survival of a patient who has non-resectable pancreatic cancer is

- (A) 6 months
- (B) 18 months
- (C) 2 to 3 years
- (D) 3 to 5 years
- (E) 5 to 10 years

12-5. MOST breast cancers are

- (A) lobular
- (B) ductal
- (C) inflammatory
- (D) other special histologies

12-6. The cumulative lifetime probability of a white female developing breast cancer is approximately

- (A) 5 percent
- (B) 12 percent
- (C) 25 percent
- (D) 33 percent

12-7. Which of the following genetic mutations have been noted to convey a markedly higher risk of breast cancer?

- (A) BRCA 1
- (B) BRCA 2
- (C) Mutation of the p53 gene
- (D) A and B only
- (E) A, B, and C

12-8. The benign breast abnormality that is MOST strongly linked with a higher subsequent risk of malignancy is

- (A) fibrocystic breast disease
- (B) fibroadenoma
- (C) fluid-filled benign cyst
- (D) hyperplasia with atypia
- (E) nipple inversion

12-9. Mammography is, generally speaking, _____ percent sensitive in the diagnosis of breast cancer.

- (A) 50
- (B) 60
- (C) 85
- (D) 95
- (E) 100

12-10. A 43-year-old woman has a palpable mass that appears negative on mammogram. The correct course of action is

(A) repeat the mammogram in 3 months
(B) repeat the mammogram in 6 months
(C) repeat the mammogram in 12 months
(D) biopsy the mass now

12-11. In general, premenopausal women with breast cancer greater than 1 cm and with negative (disease-free) nodes are

(A) treated with lumpectomy and radiation or mastectomy only
(B) treated with lumpectomy and radiation or mastectomy, followed by adjuvant chemotherapy
(C) treated with lumpectomy and radiation or mastectomy, followed by treatment with tamoxifen orally
(D) treated best with mastectomy, since it is somewhat better than local treatment with lumpectomy and radiation
(E) treated best with a radical mastectomy plus adjuvant, dose-intensive chemotherapy plus bone marrow transplant

12-12. Screening mammography

(A) should include a baseline mammogram at age 35
(B) clearly benefits women over age 50
(C) clearly benefits women over age 40
(D) should be used adjunctively with self-breast exams and provider breast exams
(E) B and D

12-13. Hodgkin's disease almost always originates in

(A) a lymph node
(B) the spleen
(C) the liver
(D) the bone marrow

12-14. A thyroid scan reveals a "cold," nonfunctional nodule. The chance of malignancy is

(A) less than 2 percent
(B) approximately 10 percent
(C) 50 percent
(D) greater than 95 percent

12-15. Known preventive measures for thyroid cancer include

(A) iodine supplements in salt
(B) avoidance of unnecessary radiation exposure
(C) obtaining routine thyroid function studies on all patients
(D) A and B
(E) A, B, and C

12-16. Patients with testicular cancer

(A) usually have pain
(B) usually have urinary tract symptoms
(C) are generally impotent
(D) are generally asymptomatic

12-17. Polyps are important to detect and treat because

(A) adenomatous polyps may develop dysplastic changes associated with colorectal malignancy
(B) polyps are precursors for diverticular disease
(C) polypoid lesions are infectious and may be spread by anal intercourse
(D) hemorrhagic GI bleeding frequently occurs with colonic polyps

12-18. Which of the following adenomatous polyps have the GREATEST potential for malignant transformation?

(A) villous adenomas
(B) tubovillous adenomas
(C) tubular adenomas
(D) none of the above

12-19. Though rare, which of the following may be an early indication of pancreatic cancer?

(A) insulin-dependent diabetes
(B) low alkaline phosphatase
(C) hypercalcemia
(D) elevated lipase
(E) low amylase

12-20. The recommended screening test(s) in the general population for colorectal cancer is/are

(A) carcinoembryonic antigen (CEA) annually over age 50
(B) annual stool tests for occult blood in persons over 50
(C) flexible sigmoidoscopy every 3 to 5 years for individuals over 50
(D) B and C
(E) all of the above

12-21. Colon cancer with nodal spread is treated with

(A) surgical resection
(B) radiation
(C) adjuvant chemotherapy with fluorouracil and levamisol
(D) A and C
(E) none of the above; palliative care only is appropriate

12-22. Rectal cancer that has spread to the lymph nodes is treated BEST with

(A) surgical resection
(B) adjuvant postoperative radiation therapy
(C) adjuvant postoperative chemotherapy
(D) A, B, and C
(E) A and B

12-23. Which of the following is the MOST common malignant neoplasm found in men?

(A) adenocarcinoma of the prostate
(B) sarcoma of the prostate
(C) squamous cell carcinoma of the prostate
(D) transitional cell carcinoma of the prostate
(E) endometrioid carcinoma of the prostate

12-24. Which of the following represents the prevalence of adenocarcinoma of the prostate?

(A) 10 percent
(B) 20 percent
(C) 30 percent
(D) 40 percent
(E) 50 percent

12-25. The incidence of cancer of the prostate is HIGHEST among which of the following ethnic groups?

(A) African-Americans
(B) Asian-Americans
(C) Mexican-Americans
(D) Native Americans
(E) Caucasian Americans

12-26. MOST oral cancers are histologically

(A) adenocystic carcinoma
(B) sarcoma
(C) basal cell carcinoma
(D) squamous cell carcinoma
(E) lymphoma

12-27. The MOST significant risk factor for the development of oral cancer is

(A) oral tobacco use
(B) heavy alcohol use
(C) betel nut chewing
(D) cigarette smoking
(E) combination of heavy alcohol and smoking

12-28. Because of the extensive lymphatic drainage system of the oral cavity, occult oral cancers may FIRST present as

(A) intraoral mass
(B) neck mass
(C) dysphagia
(D) odynophagia
(E) halitosis

12-29. The MOST common site of oral cancer is

(A) lips
(B) buccal mucosa
(C) anterior two-thirds of tongue
(D) retromolar trigone
(E) floor of mouth

12-30. Which of the following patients is MOST likely to develop an esophageal carcinoma?

(A) A 42-year-old Middle Eastern woman
(B) A 24-year-old Caucasian female smoker
(C) A 53-year-old grocer of Japanese descent
(D) A 65-year-old male coal worker in England
(E) A 36-year-old male with recurrent Barrett's esophagitis

12-31. Which of the following is the MOST common site for squamous cell carcinoma of the esophagus to develop?

(A) upper esophageal sphincter
(B) lower esophageal sphincter
(C) proximal esophagus
(D) middle esophagus
(E) distal esophagus

12-32. Which of the following is NOT considered a risk factor for the development of esophageal carcinoma?

(A) alcohol abuse
(B) ingestion of lye
(C) tobacco abuse
(D) Zenker's diverticulum
(E) Plummer-Vinson syndrome

12-33. A 45-year-old man is seen with 4 weeks of progressive dysphagia that now includes semisolids. He is having constant chest discomfort and cough and has noted a 20-lb weight loss in the last 6 weeks. A chronic smoker and a 6-pack-a-week drinker, he has no other significant health problems. Which of the following is the BEST initial diagnostic study?

(A) MRI
(B) barium swallow
(C) CT of the chest
(D) esophagogastroduodenoscopy (EGD)
(E) endoscopic retrograde cholangio-pancreatography (ERCP)

12-34. Which of the following laboratory findings is common in a patient with an esophageal carcinoma?

(A) acidosis
(B) hypoglycemia
(C) hypercalcemia
(D) markedly elevated AST
(E) macrocytic, hyperchromic anemia

12-35. Which of the following is NOT a source of structural dysphagia?

(A) scleroderma
(B) Chagas disease
(C) Zenker's diverticulum
(D) mediastinal lymphadenopathy
(E) prolonged NG tube placement

12-36. Which of the following factors increases a woman's risk of developing ovarian cancer?

(A) a history of infertility
(B) use of oral contraceptives
(C) breast feeding
(D) more than one full-term pregnancy

12-37. MOST women who present with early-stage ovarian cancer have which of the following symptoms?

(A) abnormal vaginal bleeding
(B) abdominal distention and severe gastrointestinal discomfort
(C) pelvic pressure and sensation of a mass
(D) nonspecific gastrointestinal complaints

12-38. Epithelial ovarian cancer can be differentiated from functional cysts and benign adnexal masses by evaluating all of the following EXCEPT

(A) characteristics of the mass on physical examination
(B) age of the patient and menopausal status
(C) CT scans and MRI imaging
(D) ultrasonographic features of the mass

12-39. The PRIMARY treatment for ovarian cancer, regardless of cell type or stage of disease, is

(A) chemotherapy
(B) cytoreduction and surgical staging
(C) radiation therapy
(D) ultrasonically directed aspiration

12-40. If you detect a palpable ovarian enlargement in an asymptomatic, postmenopausal woman during routine examination, which of the following is the MOST appropriate management?

(A) take a Pap smear and follow up in 6 weeks
(B) treat the patient with oral contraceptives for 6 months before reevaluating
(C) obtain serum tumor marker (CA 125) to screen for malignancy
(D) obtain a pelvic or transvaginal ultrasound and consider referring for surgical evaluation

12. ONCOLOGY

ANSWERS

12-1. The correct answer is B. Breast cancer is virtually tied with lung cancer as being the most common cause of cancer death in women. Cancer of the colon and/or rectum can be successfully treated if discovered early. Prostate cancer occurs only in men. [Kelly P: Lung cancer, in Moser RL (ed): *Primary Care for Physician Assistants*. New York, McGraw-Hill, 1998, chap 13–6.]

12-2. The correct answer is D. Any "non–small cell" carcinoma, including large cell carcinoma, squamous cell carcinoma, and adenocarcinoma, is relatively resistant to chemotherapy. Small cell carcinoma is exquisitely sensitive to chemotherapy but invariably relapses in approximately 2 years or less. [Kelly P: Lung cancer, in Moser RL (ed): *Primary Care for Physician Assistants*. New York, McGraw-Hill, 1998, chap 13–6.]

12-3. The correct answer is B. African-Americans have an increased incidence of 15 per 100,000. Caucasians, Hispanics, males, and females have an incidence rate of 9 per 100,000. [Kelly P: Pancreatic cancer, in Moser RL (ed): *Primary Care for Physician Assistants*. New York, McGraw-Hill, 1998, chap 13–8.]

12-4. The correct answer is A. Pancreatic cancer is an extremely aggressive and deadly disease. Even patients with resectable disease who undergo surgery have a 5-year survival rate of less than 25 percent. [Kelly P: Pancreatic cancer, in Moser RL (ed): *Primary Care for Physician Assistants*. New York, McGraw-Hill, 1998, chap 13–8.]

12-5. The correct answer is B. Inflammatory lesions account for 1 percent of breast cancers, and lobular lesions are found in 9 percent of breast cancers. Special histologies are found approximately 12 percent of the time. [Kelly P: Breast cancer, in Moser RL (ed): *Primary Care for Physician Assistants*. New York, McGraw-Hill, 1998, chap 13–4.]

12-6. The correct answer is B. It is generally acknowledged that the cumulative lifetime probability of developing breast cancer is 12 percent and of dying from breast cancer, 3.5 percent. [Kelly P: Breast cancer, in Moser RL (ed): *Primary Care for Physician Assistants*. New York, McGraw-Hill, 1998, chap 13–4.]

12-7. The correct answer is E. BRCA 1, BRCA 2, and mutations of the p53 gene all convey a markedly increased risk of breast cancer. [Kelly P: Breast cancer, in Moser RL (ed): *Primary Care for Physician Assistants*. New York, McGraw-Hill, 1998, chap 13–4.]

12-8. The correct answer is D. "Fibrocystic breast disease" is a "garbage can," nonhistologic diagnosis and is not meaningful in determining risk of breast cancer in the future. Fibroadenomas, fluid-filled cysts, and chronic nipple inversion (as opposed to new-onset nipple inversion unilaterally) do not herald breast cancer risk. [Kelly P: Breast cancer, in Moser RL (ed): *Primary Care for Physician Assistants*. New York, McGraw-Hill, 1998, chap 13–4.]

12-9. **The correct answer is C.** Mammography is a good test, though less sensitive in younger women. Few tests are 100 percent sensitive, and radiologic imaging must always be correlated with clinical impression. [Kelly P: Breast cancer, in Moser RL (ed): *Primary Care for Physician Assistants*. New York, McGraw-Hill, 1998, chap 13–4.]

12-10. **The correct answer is D.** A palpable mass that is negative on mammography should be biopsied. Failure to biopsy is a leading cause of malpractice litigation. [Kelly P: Breast cancer, in Moser RL (ed): *Primary Care for Physician Assistants*. New York, McGraw-Hill, 1998, chap 13–4.]

12-11. **The correct answer is B.** Lumpectomy and radiation are equivalent to mastectomy for smaller masses. Women with masses over 1 cm who are premenopausal are best protected with adjuvant chemotherapy. [Kelly P: Breast cancer, in Moser RL (ed): *Primary Care for Physician Assistants*. New York, McGraw-Hill, 1998, chap 13–4.]

12-12. **The correct answer is E.** An important part of breast screening includes provider and patient breast examination. Screening women between the ages of 40 and 50 with mammography is controversial because of the *relatively* low prevalence in this age group, the large number of false-positive mammograms in women between 40 and 50, and the huge financial and emotional cost of positive screening mammograms and subsequent biopsies that reveal benign disease. [Kelly P: Breast cancer, in Moser RL (ed): *Primary Care for Physician Assistants*. New York, McGraw-Hill, 1998, chap 13–4.]

12-13. **The correct answer is A.** Hodgkin's disease almost always originates in a lymph node. The axial lymphatic system is almost always affected; involvement of peripheral nodes outside of the cervical chain is less common. Hodgkin's demonstrates contiguous progression throughout lymphatic tissue. An extranodal site is frequently the spleen; other extranodal sites are rare at the time of disease presentation, but can include the liver and bone marrow. [Kelly P: Hodgkin's disease, in Moser RL (ed): *Primary Care for Physician Assistants*. New York, McGraw-Hill, 1998, chap 13–11.]

12-14. **The correct answer is B.** Approximately 10 percent of nonfunctional, "cold" nodules seen on thyroid scans will be malignant. [Kelly P: Thyroid cancer, in Moser RL (ed): *Primary Care for Physician Assistants*. New York, McGraw-Hill, 1998, chap 13–10.]

12-15. **The correct answer is D.** Persons that have been exposed to excess radiation and persons who have suffered iodine deprivation are at higher risk for thyroid cancer. Thyroid function tests neither prevent nor screen for thyroid cancer. [Kelly P: Thyroid cancer, in Moser RL (ed): *Primary Care for Physician Assistants*. New York, McGraw-Hill, 1998, chap 13–10.]

12-16. **The correct answer is D.** Patients with testicular cancer are asymptomatic over 50 percent of the time. [Kelly P: Testicular cancer, in Moser RL (ed): *Primary Care for Physician Assistants*. New York, McGraw-Hill, 1998, chap 13–9.]

12-17. **The correct answer is A.** Polyps are not infectious lesions and have no direct correlation to the formation of diverticula of the colon. Colorectal polyps are significant because it is believed that most cases of adenocarcinoma of the colon arise in adenomatous polyps. Approximately 25 percent of polyps are adenomatous by histologic report, with 3 to 5 percent of adenomas found to have malignant changes. [Kelly P: Colorectal cancer, in Moser RL (ed): *Primary Care for Physician Assistants*. New York, McGraw-Hill, 1998, chap 13–5.]

12-18. **The correct answer is A.** Villous adenomas have the greatest potential for malignant transformation (>50 percent) and tubular adenomas the least. [Kelly P: Colorectal cancer, in Moser RL (ed): *Primary Care for Physician Assistants*. New York, McGraw-Hill, 1998, chap 13–5.]

12-19. **The correct answer is A.** Since pancreatic cancer is common in the elderly the sudden development of IDDM is quite unusual and should trigger a full investigation. The elderly are much more likely to develop progressive NIDDM. Pancreatic cancer is likely to cause hypocalcemia, hyperbilirubinemia, and elevated ALT and alkaline phosphates—but these are usually late findings. [Kelly P: Pancreatic cancer, in Moser RL (ed): *Primary Care for Physician Assistants.* New York, McGraw-Hill, 1998, chap 13–8.]

12-20. **The correct answer is D.** Currently, the CEA is not recommended as a screening test. Annual tests for occult blood and interval flexible sigmoidoscopy are recommended by the American Cancer Society for individuals over 50 without other known risk factors. [Kelly P: Colorectal cancer, in Moser RL (ed): *Primary Care for Physician Assistants.* New York, McGraw-Hill, 1998, chap 13–5.]

12-21. **The correct answer is D.** Colon cancer with nodal spread is treated with initial surgery with curative intent, then with adjuvant fluorouracil and levamisole in various dosing schemes for up to 1 year. Three large, prospective, randomized trials have demonstrated that adjuvant therapy improves the 5-year survival rate approximately 10 to 15 percent. [Kelly P: Colorectal cancer, in Moser RL (ed): *Primary Care for Physician Assistants.* New York, McGraw-Hill, 1998, chap 13–5.]

12-22. **The correct answer is D.** Rectal cancer is almost always treated postsurgically with adjuvant radiation therapy and concomitant fluorouracil. After the completion of combination radiation therapy and chemotherapy, adjuvant therapy with fluorouracil and levamisole is indicated for disease that has spread locally or to adjacent nodes. This aggressive treatment is necessary because of the technical difficulty of achieving adequate clear surgical margins after resection of rectal cancer. [Kelly P: Colorectal cancer, in Moser RL (ed): *Primary Care for Physician Assistants.* New York, McGraw-Hill, 1998, chap 13–5.]

12-23. **The correct answer is A.** Adenocarcinoma of the prostate is the most common malignant neoplasm found in men. It accounts for 33 percent of all cancers diagnosed in men. Adjusted for age, 80 percent of all cases of cancer of the prostate are diagnosed in men over 65. [Mosier WA: Prostate cancer, in Moser RL (ed): *Primary Care for Physician Assistants.* New York, McGraw-Hill, 1998, chap 13–2.]

12-24. **The correct answer is C.** As stated in Answer 12-23 (above), adenocarcinoma of the prostate is the most common malignant neoplasm found in men. It accounts for 33 percent of all cancers diagnosed in men. The risk of acquiring cancer of the prostate increases with age. It is the second most commonly occurring cancer in American men over the age of 65. [Mosier WA: Prostate cancer, in Moser RL (ed): *Primary Care for Physician Assistants.* New York, McGraw-Hill, 1998, chap 13–2.]

12-25. **The correct answer is A.** For an unknown reason, the incidence of cancer of the prostate is highest among African-American men, in spite of the fact that cancer of the prostate is considered rare in Africa. The incidence of this cancer is lowest among Asians. Although the etiology is unknown, cancer of the prostate is more common in men who have had a first-degree relative diagnosed with the disease. [Mosier WA: Prostate cancer, in Moser RL (ed): *Primary Care for Physician Assistants.* New York, McGraw-Hill, 1998, chap 13–2.]

12-26. **The correct answer is D.** Approximately 90 percent of all oral cancers are histologically squamous cell carcinomas. Sarcoma, lymphoma, and adenocystic carcinoma are rare and are included in the remaining 10 percent of all other cell types demonstrated in histologic studies of oral cancer tumors. Basal cell carcinoma is the most common skin cancer about the head and neck. [Dobbs KJ: Oral cancer, in Moser RL (ed): *Primary Care for Physician Assistants.* New York, McGraw-Hill, 1998, chap 13-3.]

12-27. The correct answer is E. Three-fourths of all oral cancers in the United States are caused by tobacco and alcohol use in combination. Smokeless tobacco, cigarette smoking, alcohol, and betel nut chewing all have been shown to increase the incidence of oral cancers, but not nearly to the degree that the combination of smoking and alcohol does. [Dobbs KJ: Oral cancer, in Moser RL (ed): *Primary Care for Physician Assistants*. New York, McGraw-Hill, 1998, chap 13-3.]

12-28. The correct answer is B. The extensive lymphatic system of the oral cavity may explain the increased rate of early metastasis in oral cancers. Any neck mass present for 1 to 2 months deserves complete evaluation to look for an occult oral cancer. Typical oral cancers are symptomatic and may present with intraoral mass, ulcerations with or without bleeding, pain, halitosis, odynophagia, dysphagia, trismus, decreased tongue mobility, loosening of teeth, or ill-fitting dentures. [Dobbs KJ: Oral cancer, in Moser RL (ed): *Primary Care for Physician Assistants*. New York, McGraw-Hill, 1998, chap 13-3.]

12-29. The correct answer is A. Cancer of the lip accounts for approximately 30 percent of all oral cancers. The lower lip is more frequently involved than the upper lip. In descending order the frequency of occurrence of the remaining oral cancers is anterior two-thirds of tongue, floor of mouth, alveolar ridge, buccal mucosa, retromolar trigone, hard palate. [Dobbs KJ: Oral cancer, in Moser RL (ed): *Primary Care for Physician Assistants*. New York, McGraw-Hill, 1998, chap 13-3.]

12-30. The correct answer is E. Esophageal carcinomas are well known in the Far East and are found primarily in men over 50 years of age. Smokers also have increased risk of developing esophageal carcinoma. But in the population given, the recurrent Barrett's esophagitis is the vital clue. Usually the result of severe GERD, Barrett's esophagitis is a significant risk factor in the development of adenocarcinoma of the esophagus. Once diagnosed, the patient is committed to a yearly esophagogastroduodenoscopy (EGD) to screen for cancer. [Heinly AP: Esophageal carcinomas, in Moser RL (ed): *Primary Care for Physician Assistants*. New York, McGraw-Hill, 1998, chap 13–1.]

12-31. The correct answer is D. Chronic irritation and inflammation of the squamous cell layer of the esophagus lends itself to carcinomas. The middle esophagus, followed by the distal esophagus, is the most common site. Persistent atypia predisposes to malignancy over time. [Heinly AP: Esophageal carcinomas, in Moser RL (ed): *Primary Care for Physician Assistants*. New York, McGraw-Hill, 1998, chap 13–1.]

12-32. The correct answer is D. Zenker's diverticulum is a mechanical problem usually associated with the upper esophagus. A diverticulum develops and can enlarge with ingested foods. It causes regurgitation and cough but it does not predispose the esophagus to cancer. Smoking, alcohol, and chemical ingestion can cause tissue disruption or decreased blood supply. The mechanism of the Plummer-Vinson syndrome is unclear but may be due to diminished oxygen delivery with its significant iron-deficiency anemia. [Heinly AP: Esophageal carcinomas, in Moser RL (ed): *Primary Care for Physician Assistants*. New York, McGraw-Hill, 1998, chap 13–1.]

12-33. The correct answer is D. All the choices, with the exception of the ERCP, are good ones to evaluate this patient for esophageal carcinoma or to determine its spread, but the best initial test is the EGD. The symptoms of progressive dysphagia, chest pain, cough, and weight loss should cause alarm bells to ring. The fastest and most definitive answers can be obtained with an EGD. If done first, the barium study may give the size and compression of a lesion, but the tissue diagnosis would have to wait several days for the barium to clear. [Heinly AP: Esophageal carcinomas, in Moser RL (ed): *Primary Care for Physician Assistants*. New York, McGraw-Hill, 1998, chap 13–1.]

12-34. **The correct answer is C.** Hypercalcemia is a common initial presentation, maybe even before dysphagia. Patients will complain of rapid onset of spreading weakness, nausea, sedation, and eventually stupor. The anemia is usually one associated with blood loss, a microcytic-hypochromic anemia. With metastasis, liver enzymes will rise, but usually not markedly. [Heinly AP: Esophageal carcinomas, in Moser RL (ed): *Primary Care for Physician Assistants*. New York, McGraw-Hill, 1998, chap 13–1.]

12-35. **The correct answer is A.** Scleroderma is a motor disorder that will cause some esophageal dysphagia or changes in up to 80 percent of scleroderma patients. The dysphagia is due to decreased or absent peristalsis. Chagas disease can cause a mega-esophagus secondary to esophageal infestation by trypanosomiasis. Zenker's diverticulum, NGT placement, and mediastinal lymphadenopathy all reflect mechanical disruptions of the esophagus that can cause dysphagia. [Heinly AP: Esophageal carcinomas, in Moser RL (ed): *Primary Care for Physician Assistants*. New York, McGraw-Hill, 1998, chap 13–1.]

12-36. **The correct answer is A.** One of the main theories related to the development of ovarian cancer is repeated ovulatory activity and incessant ovulation. Supporting this hypothesis, the use of oral contraceptives, multiparity, and a history of breast feeding have been shown to offer a protective benefit against ovarian cancer by reducing the amount of insult to the ovarian surface during a woman's lifetime. Genetic factors are also associated with the development of this disease. Women with a negative family history of ovarian cancer have a lifetime risk of 1 in 70. Conversely, a woman with one first-degree relative with ovarian cancer is at a 5 percent risk, and two or more relatives raises the risk to 7 percent. [Naccarto-Coleman A: Ovarian cancer, in Moser RL (ed): *Primary Care for Physician Assistants*. New York, McGraw-Hill, 1998, chap 13–7.]

12-37. **The correct answer is D.** Ovarian cancer develops insidiously and with few, if any, symptoms in the early stages. At the time of diagnosis, most patients are asymptomatic or have nonspecific complaints such as nausea, dyspepsia, and altered bowel habits. As the disease progresses, the symptoms become more intense and specific. This is related to the enlarging pelvic mass and increased abdominal girth secondary to ascites. [Naccarto-Coleman A: Ovarian cancer, in Moser RL (ed): *Primary Care for Physician Assistants*. New York, McGraw-Hill, 1998, chap 13–7.]

12-38. **The correct answer is C.** Ultrasound, especially transvaginal sonography, is extremely useful in evaluating pelvic masses. The size, complexity, morphology, and likelihood of malignancy can generally be estimated from performing this procedure. Extensive imaging studies, such as the CT scan and MRI, are reserved for select cases only. They provide very little additional information and are not cost effective. Transvaginal ultrasounds are the most efficient, accurate, and cost-effective methods in evaluating a pelvic mass. [Naccarto-Coleman A: Ovarian cancer, in Moser RL (ed): *Primary Care for Physician Assistants*. New York, McGraw-Hill, 1998, chap 13–7.]

12-39. **The correct answer is B.** Chemotherapy is the main treatment following surgical cytoreduction and debulking of the tumor. Used alone, it is ineffective in reducing or eliminating the tumor. Radiation therapy has a limited role because of the side effects involved in treating the entire abdominal area. Ultrasonically directed cyst aspiration is not recommended because of its high recurrence rate and poor diagnostic capabilities. Aggressive debulking and accurate surgical staging are paramount in the prognosis and treatment of this disease. [Naccarto-Coleman A: Ovarian cancer, in Moser RL (ed): *Primary Care for Physician Assistants*. New York, McGraw-Hill, 1998, chap 13–7.]

12-40. **The correct answer is D.** Ovarian atrophy generally ensues within 1 or 2 years after reaching menopause. Therefore, an enlarged, palpable ovary in a postmenopausal woman is considered abnormal and warrants surgical exploration. Further characterization of the ovary can be achieved by obtaining a pelvic ultrasound. Pap smear may occasionally reveal malignant ovarian cells, but it is not considered a reliable screening test for ovarian carcinoma. Tumor markers have limited specificity and are not recommended as a screening method for ovarian cancer. They are predominantly used to monitor the disease after a diagnosis has been established. Oral contraceptives are indicated in the treatment of nonneoplastic ovarian disorders predominantly found in women who are premenopausal and in their reproductive years. [Naccarto-Coleman A: Ovarian cancer, in Moser RL (ed): *Primary Care for Physician Assistants*. New York, McGraw-Hill, 1998, chap 13–7.]

SECTION 13
OPHTHALMOLOGY

13. OPHTHALMOLOGY

QUESTIONS

DIRECTIONS: Each question below contains suggested responses. Choose the **one** **best** response to each question.

13-1. An acute infection of the glands of Zeis or Moll around the eyelashes, left untreated, may lead to

(A) acute dacryocystitis
(B) preseptal cellulitis
(C) orbital cellulitis
(D) seborrheic blepharitis
(E) conjunctivitis

13-2. The inward turning of the eyelid, common in aging, is called

(A) entropion
(B) coloboma
(C) epicanthus
(D) hordeolum

13-3. Which cranial nerve would be the cause of ectropion in facial nerve palsy?

(A) CN V
(B) CN VI
(C) CN VII
(D) CN III

13-4. Your patient complains of a palpable, well-defined subcutaneous nodule within the upper eyelid. Exam reveals a blocked meibomian gland of the upper lid with swelling and mild redness. INITIAL treatment would consist of which of the following?

(A) warm compresses and massage over the lesion
(B) steroid injection into the lesion
(C) lubrication of the affected eye with artificial tears
(D) incision and curettage of the lesion
(E) systemic antibiotics

13-5. A 30-year-old man presents to the primary care clinic with a 1-day history of unilateral conjunctival redness and irritation, a mucoid discharge, and eye pain with mild photophobia. He denies any trauma. On physical exam, you notice an acutely red eye with discharge and tearing. Small vesicles were noted on the eyelid and lid margins. A slit-lamp examination after fluorescein dye shows multiple corneal ulcers, and some that form branching epithelial (dendritic) ulcers. Your patient MOST likely has

(A) chlamydial conjunctivitis
(B) Sjögren's syndrome
(C) hyperacute bacterial conjunctivitis secondary to *Neisseria gonorrhoeae*
(D) herpes simplex viral (HSV) conjunctivitis
(E) monilial conjunctivitis secondary to HIV infection

13-6. Topical ophthalmic corticosteroids are indicated for inflammatory conditions of the eye for all of the following conditions EXCEPT

(A) allergic conjunctivitis
(B) herpes simplex keratitis
(C) uveitis
(D) episcleritis

13-7. What is the MOST common causative agent for conjunctivitis?

(A) *Staphylococcus aureus*
(B) *Streptococcus pneumoniae*
(C) viruses
(D) *Haemophilus influenzae*

13-8. Which symptom listed below can indicate that there is corneal involvement in conjunctivitis?

(A) hyperemia
(B) photophobia
(C) pruritus
(D) periocular edema

13-9. Which topical antibiotic medication is often used instead of silver nitrate for the prophylaxis of ophthalmia neonatorum?

(A) neomycin ointment
(B) bacitracin with polymyxin B ointment
(C) erythromycin ointment 0.5%
(D) gentamycin ointment

13-10. In diabetic retinopathy, all of the following symptoms would require an immediate referral to an eye doctor EXCEPT

(A) initial diagnosis of type I diabetes mellitus (DM)
(B) new onset of floaters
(C) sudden decrease of vision
(D) flashes of light

13-11. What is the LEADING cause of blindness among working-aged adults in the United States?

(A) central retinal artery occlusion (CRAO)
(B) acute ocular trauma
(C) diabetic retinopathy
(D) retinoblastoma

13-12. All of the following are symptoms of acute uveitis EXCEPT

(A) pain
(B) redness
(C) photophobia
(D) profuse tearing

13-13. Retinopathy of prematurity (ROP) is a condition of premature babies that is almost always caused by

(A) high PaO_2
(B) high FiO_2
(C) high $PaCO_2$
(D) high $FiCO_2$

13-14. All of the following conditions present with defects of the red reflex EXCEPT

(A) retinoblastoma
(B) congenital cataract
(C) persistent hyperplastic primary vitreous (PHPV)
(D) retinopathy of prematurity (ROP)

13-15. The MOST common cause of vitreous hemorrhage is

(A) hypertension
(B) diabetic retinopathy
(C) sickle cell disease
(D) vascular occlusion of the eye

13-16. Which of the below objective clinical findings makes the diagnosis of anterior ischemic optic neuropathy (AION)?

(A) increased visual acuity
(B) an afferent pupil defect
(C) a dense central scotoma
(D) a pale swollen nerve with vision loss

13-17. A finding during ophthalmoscopy of a "blood and thunder" fundus is unique to the diagnosis of

(A) central retinal artery occlusion (CRAO)
(B) central retinal vein occlusion (CRVO)
(C) anterior ischemic vein occlusion
(D) vitreous hemorrhage

13-18. What is MOST likely the etiology for sudden loss of vision when there is no apparent cause?

(A) vascular compromise
(B) infection
(C) retinal detachment
(D) neurologic degeneration

13-19. A common side effect after using scopolamine 0.25% drops to reduce the risk of iritis in the treatment of foreign bodies and corneal abrasions is

(A) pain due to ciliary muscle spasm
(B) epithelial disruption
(C) constricted pupil
(D) dilated pupil

13-20. The HALLMARK symptom of a foreign body or corneal abrasion is

(A) acute pain
(B) photophobia
(C) hyperemia
(D) profuse tearing

13-21. What is the MOST common symptom of late-onset strabismus caused by trauma, stroke, or tumor?

(A) loss of vision in the affected eye
(B) unilateral blurred vision
(C) diplopia
(D) hyphema

13-22. A 44-year-old, previously healthy male presents with a sudden onset of fever, acute pain and warmth around the eyes, diffuse lid swelling, decreased vision, and double vision. Prior history indicates moderate to severe infraorbital pain for the past 3 days associated with the patient's seasonal allergies. Of the following, the MOST appropriate INITIAL diagnosis would be

(A) orbital cellulitis
(B) conjunctivitis
(C) uveitis
(D) herpes simplex keratitis

13-23. The etiology of insult for a subconjunctival hemorrhage would include all of the following EXCEPT

(A) trauma
(B) Valsalva maneuvers
(C) bleeding disorders
(D) hypotension

13-24. A 35-year-old female with a history of severe chronic blepharitis presents with a complaint of sudden onset of left eye pain since awakening this morning. Examination reveals a corneal ulceration. The preferred course of action is

(A) referral to an ophthalmologist
(B) steroid eye drops
(C) artificial tears
(D) warm compresses and eye patch

13-25. All of the following are appropriate treatments for blepharitis EXCEPT

(A) warm compresses to eyelid margins
(B) lid scrubs on a regular basis
(C) artificial tears
(D) steroid eyedrops

13-26. The infectious agent commonly associated with blepharitis is

(A) streptococcal organisms
(B) staphylococcal organisms
(C) *Haemophilus influenzae*
(D) enterococcal organisms

13-27. The microorganism MOST commonly associated with orbital cellulitis in children under 5 years old is

(A) *Staphylococcus*
(B) *Streptococcus*
(C) *Pseudomonas*
(D) *Haemophilus influenzae*

13-28. A 44-year-old male presents with ocular pain of acute onset, decreased vision, haloes around lights, and nausea. The intraocular pressure is greater than 40 mmHg, the conjunctiva is injected, the cornea is cloudy, and the pupil is in the mid-dilated position and minimally reactive. Visual acuity is reduced. You suspect

(A) cataract
(B) open-angle glaucoma
(C) herpes simplex keratitis
(D) angle-closure glaucoma

13-29. Intraocular pressure diagnostic of glaucoma must be greater than

(A) 19 mmHg
(B) 20 mmHg
(C) 21 mmHg
(D) 22 mmHg

13-30. A 59-year-old male presents with complaints of central vision loss. His visual acuity on last examination at the health fair had changed from 20/200 to 20/400. He states that he does get around well by seeing things on the "sides" of his eyes. Your examination shows scattered yellow deposits in the macular area with pigment atrophy and clumping. You suspect

(A) diabetic retinopathy
(B) anterior ischemic optic neuropathy
(C) dry age-related macular degeneration
(D) wet age-related macular degeneration

13. OPHTHALMOLOGY

ANSWERS

13-1. The correct answer is B. Hordeolum (usually caused by *Staphylococcus aureus* abscesses of the meibomian gland) may lead to diffuse superficial lid infection known as "preseptal cellulitis." Dacryocystitis is infection of the lacrimal sac. Orbital cellulitis is an infection that enters the orbit either directly through the sinuses or by circulation. Seborrheic blepharitis is a chronic inflammation of the lid margin. Conjunctivitis affects the conjunctival lining of the eye. [Warnimont S: Chalazion and hordeolum (stye), in Moser RL (ed): *Primary Care for Physician Assistants*. New York, McGraw-Hill, 1998, chap 14–15.]

13-2. The correct answer is A. The inward turning of the eyelid always affects the lower lid and is partly the result of laxity of the lower lid retractors. [Ota WT, Sousa FJ: Entropion and ectropion, in Moser RL (ed): *Primary Care for Physician Assistants*. New York, McGraw-Hill, 1998, chap 14–9.]

13-3. The correct answer is C. The facial cranial nerve (VII) is the cause of ectropion in facial nerve palsy. The other cranial nerve choices are incorrect. [Ota WT, Sousa FJ: Entropion and ectropion, in Moser RL (ed): *Primary Care for Physician Assistants*. New York, McGraw-Hill, 1998, chap 14–9.]

13-4. The correct answer is A. Initial conservative treatment of this chalazion includes warm compresses for 15 to 20 minutes 4 times per day, light massage over the lesion, and perhaps use of a *topical* antibiotic such as bacitracin or erythromycin ointment 2 times per day. Incision and curettage or steroid injection may be considered if the lesion persists beyond 3 to 4 weeks. Lubrication with artificial tears and systemic antibiotics are not necessary. [Warnimont S: Chalazion and hordeolum (stye), in Moser RL (ed): *Primary Care for Physician Assistants*. New York, McGraw-Hill, 1998, chap 14–15.]

13-5. The correct answer is D. The presence of discrete or multiple branching dendritic ulcers is characteristic of herpetic involvement of the eye. Herpetic vesicles are also common on the eyelid and eye margins and may be associated with edema. [Ota WT, Sousa FJ: Herpes simplex keratitis, in Moser RL (ed): *Primary Care for Physician Assistants*. New York, McGraw-Hill, 1998, chap 14–10.]

13-6. The correct answer is B. Steroids enhance the activity of the herpesvirus and perforation of the cornea may occur. Any patient receiving local ocular corticosteroid therapy should be under the collaborative care of an ophthalmologist. [Ota WT, Sousa FJ: Herpes simplex keratitis, in Moser RL (ed): *Primary Care for Physician Assistants*. New York, McGraw-Hill, 1998, chap 14–10.]

13-7. The correct answer is C. *S. aureus, S. pneumoniae,* and *H. influenzae* are all common bacterial causes of conjunctivitis, but nonspecific viruses remain the most common cause. [Ota WT, Sousa FJ: Conjunctivitis, in Moser RL (ed): *Primary Care for Physician Assistants*. New York, McGraw-Hill, 1998, chap 14–16.]

13-8. The correct answer is B. Photophobia can occur in conjunctivitis when there is corneal involvement. Pruritus is a hallmark for allergic conjunctivitis. [Ota WT, Sousa FJ: Conjunctivitis, in Moser RL (ed): *Primary Care for Physician Assistants*. New York, McGraw-Hill, 1998, chap 14–16.]

13-9. **The correct answer is C.** Erythromycin ophthalmic ointment is an effective substitution and produces less chemical conjunctivitis. [Ota WT, Sousa FJ: Conjunctivitis, in Moser RL (ed): *Primary Care for Physician Assistants.* New York, McGraw-Hill, 1998, chap 14–16.]

13-10. **The correct answer is A.** Retinal evaluation for type I DM is recommended 5 years after diagnosis. [Ota WT, Sousa FJ: Diabetic retinopathy, in Moser RL (ed): *Primary Care for Physician Assistants.* New York, McGraw-Hill, 1998, chap 14–8.]

13-11. **The correct answer is D.** The risk of blindness increases with the duration of diabetic retinopathy and the patient's age. Retinoblastoma is a leading cause of blindness in infants. [Ota WT, Sousa FJ: Diabetic retinopathy, in Moser RL (ed): *Primary Care for Physician Assistants.* New York, McGraw-Hill, 1998, chap 14–8.]

13-12. **The correct answer is D.** The classic triad of signs and symptoms of acute uveitis is redness, pain, and photophobia. [Ota WT, Sousa FJ: Uveitis, in Moser RL (ed): *Primary Care for Physician Assistants.* New York, McGraw-Hill, 1998, chap 14–2.]

13-13. **The correct answer is B.** ROP is a condition of premature babies who have almost always been on high FiO_2 due to abnormal pulmonary development. Occasionally ROP can develop with high PaO_2 and a normal FiO_2. [Ota WT, Sousa FJ: Leukocoria, in Moser RL (ed): *Primary Care for Physician Assistants.* New York, McGraw-Hill, 1998, chap 14–11.]

13-14. **The correct answer is A.** Retinoblastoma is the most common malignant intraocular tumor in children. The most common presenting findings of retinoblastoma are leukocoria (white-pupil) and/or strabismus. [Ota WT, Sousa FJ: Leukocoria, in Moser RL (ed): *Primary Care for Physician Assistants.* New York, McGraw-Hill, 1998, chap 14–11.]

13-15. **The correct answer is B.** Diabetes mellitus is the most common cause of a vitreous hemorrhage. Hypertension, sickle cell anemia, and vascular occlusions are all diagnostic considerations with vitreous hemorrhage. [Ota WT, Sousa FJ: Diabetic retinopathy, in Moser RL (ed): *Primary Care for Physician Assistants.* New York, McGraw-Hill, 1998, chap 14–8.]

13-16. **The correct answer is D.** In AION the optic nerve is swollen, showing blurred disc margins with a very small or no cup. The vessels on or near the nerve are obscured, which results in pallor of the nerve. [Ota WT, Sousa FJ: Sudden visual loss in one eye, in Moser RL (ed): *Primary Care for Physician Assistants.* New York, McGraw-Hill, 1998, chap 14–14.]

13-17. **The correct answer is B.** CRVO's most dramatic clinical objective finding is diffuse hemorrhages throughout the retina during fundoscopy. Because of the dramatic appearance of the hemorrhages, the fundus is described as "blood and thunder." [Ota WT, Sousa FJ: Sudden visual loss in one eye, in Moser RL (ed): *Primary Care for Physician Assistants.* New York, McGraw-Hill, 1998, chap 14–14.]

13-18. **The correct answer is A.** Vascular compromise is almost always the etiology when any vision loss occurs suddenly and for no apparent reason. [Ota WT, Sousa FJ: Sudden visual loss in one eye, in Moser RL (ed): *Primary Care for Physician Assistants.* New York, McGraw-Hill, 1998, chap 14–14.]

13-19. **The correct answer is D.** Pupillary dilation results from paralysis of the ciliary muscle with use of a cycloplegic medication. [Ota WT, Sousa FJ: Corneal abrasion and foreign body, in Moser RL (ed): *Primary Care for Physician Assistants.* New York, McGraw-Hill, 1998, chap 14–7.]

13-20. **The correct answer is A.** Due to the abundant pain receptors from CN V, acute pain is the hallmark symptom. Photophobia, hyperemia, and profuse tearing are also symptoms found in foreign bodies and corneal abrasions but can be found in several other conditions. [Ota WT, Sousa FJ: Corneal abrasion and foreign body, in Moser RL (ed): *Primary Care for Physician Assistants.* New York, McGraw-Hill, 1998, chap 14–7.]

13-21. **The correct answer is C.** Diplopia is often the result of late-onset strabismus. The treatment goal is reducing the double vision. [Ota WT, Sousa FJ: Strabismus, in Moser RL (ed): *Primary Care for Physician Assistants.* New York, McGraw-Hill, 1998, chap 14–12.]

13-22. **The correct answer is A.** This patient presents with symptoms of a paraorbital sinusitis that has progressed to the common symptoms of acute pain, warmth around eyes, decreased and double vision, diffuse lid swelling, and fever associated with a history of paranasal sinusitis (the most common cause) that make up the diagnosis of orbital cellulitis. [Ota WT, Sousa FJ: Orbital cellulitis, in Moser RL (ed): *Primary Care for Physician Assistants.* New York, McGraw-Hill, 1998, chap 14–6.]

13-23. **The correct answer is D.** *Hyper*tension can be a cause in subconjunctival hemorrhage, but not hypotension. An evaluation of blood pressure is indicated on all patients presenting with nontraumatic hemorrhage. [Ota WT, Sousa FJ: Subconjunctival hemorrhage, in Moser RL (ed): *Primary Care for Physician Assistants.* New York, McGraw-Hill, 1998, chap 14–13.]

13-24. **The correct answer is A.** This patient should be referred to an ophthalmologist. Corneal ulcerations in severe blepharitis that can impair vision are considered a red flag for this disease. Steroids should not be considered for the treatment of blepharitis. Artificial tears and warm compresses will treat the blepharitis but not the corneal ulceration. [Ota WT, Sousa FJ: Blepharitis, in Moser RL (ed): *Primary Care for Physician Assistants.* New York, McGraw-Hill, 1998, chap 14–5.]

13-25. **The correct answer is D.** Steroids should not be considered as part of the treatment plan for blepharitis due to the potential for serious complications if they are used inappropriately. [Ota WT, Sousa FJ: Blepharitis, in Moser RL (ed): *Primary Care for Physician Assistants.* New York, McGraw-Hill, 1998, chap 14–5.]

13-26. **The correct answer is B.** *S. aureus* and *S. epidermis* are the most common organisms that cause blepharitis. [Ota WT, Sousa FJ: Blepharitis, in Moser RL (ed): *Primary Care for Physician Assistants.* New York, McGraw-Hill, 1998, chap 14–5.]

13-27. **The correct answer is D.** *Haemophilus influenzae* is the most commonly involved organism in orbital cellulitis and is exclusively found in children under 5 years old. [Ota WT, Sousa FJ: Orbital cellulitis, in Moser RL (ed): *Primary Care for Physician Assistants.* New York, McGraw-Hill, 1998, chap 14–6.]

13-28. **The correct answer is D.** Angle-closure glaucoma tends to have acute episodes with the symptoms described. Open-angle glaucoma is asymptomatic until very late in the process. [Ota WT, Sousa FJ: Glaucoma, in Moser RL (ed): *Primary Care for Physician Assistants.* New York, McGraw-Hill, 1998, chap 14–1.]

13-29. **The correct answer is C.** An intraocular pressure greater than 21 mmHg is normally present in glaucoma (but not always). [Ota WT, Sousa FJ: Glaucoma, in Moser RL (ed): *Primary Care for Physician Assistants.* New York, McGraw-Hill, 1998, chap 14–1.]

13-30. **The correct answer is C.** Age-related macular degeneration is one of the leading causes of new blindness in older adults. It involves central vision (visual acuity) and is bilateral and often asymmetric. [Ota WT, Sousa FJ: Age-related macular degeneration, in Moser RL (ed): *Primary Care for Physician Assistants.* New York, McGraw-Hill, 1998, chap 14–3.]

SECTION 14
PEDIATRICS

14. PEDIATRICS

QUESTIONS

DIRECTIONS: Each question below contains suggested responses. Choose the **one best** response to each question.

14-1. Which of the following social skills would be expected to be accomplished by age 3 years?

(A) engages in parallel play
(B) engages in interactive play
(C) dresses self completely
(D) bathes self skillfully

14-2. By which age would you expect the following: Language is well established, conversation is mature, five-word sentences are used, and a large vocabulary is demonstrated?

(A) 1 year
(B) 2 years
(C) 3 years
(D) 4 years

14-3. A 12-month-old child presents to your office for a routine exam. You expect that this child would have accomplished which of the following developmental milestones?

(A) jumps down from low object
(B) walks when led with support
(C) throws ball and catches with assistance
(D) rides a tricycle

14-4. Which of the following descriptions accurately defines the Moro reflex?

(A) elicited in response to touching the cheek and results in turning of the head and opening the mouth
(B) occurs when an object is placed in the infant's hand causing the infant to tightly grasp the object
(C) occurs when the bottom of the foot is stroked and the toes fan outward in response
(D) occurs when the neck and limbs contract in response to allowing the infant's head to fall backward suddenly

14-5. Which of the following is an indication that a child should be referred for further evaluation for possible delayed language development?

(A) failure to speak intelligibly 90 percent of the time by age 2
(B) failure to babble by age 9 months
(C) stuttering at age 2
(D) all of the above

14-6. A family has a history of hypercholesterolemia in both parents. The best advice to offer about proper diet for their preschool children would be

(A) No dietary restrictions are needed as this will inhibit growth.
(B) Children naturally eat what is best for their needs.
(C) High-fat diets in prepubescent children are not related to risk of adult heart disease.
(D) Total daily fat intake should be limited to about 30 percent of daily calorie intake.
(E) No concern is needed until age 21.

14-7. Infants who have been fed whole cow's milk only are likely to present with

(A) childhood obesity
(B) frequent otitis media
(C) multiple allergies
(D) iron-deficiency anemia
(E) constipation

14-8. Specific characteristics of a premature infant include all EXCEPT

(A) less than 2500 g (5.5 lb) weight
(B) less than 270 days gestation
(C) less than 8 h of maternal labor
(D) more water/less protein per kilogram of body weight
(E) weak neuromuscular system, causing difficulty sucking

14-9. Breast milk and infant formulas are comparable in nutritional value except breast milk provides

(A) a higher protein level
(B) no fluoride protection
(C) adequate iron content
(D) good vitamin K protection
(E) overprotection from vitamin D

14-10. Which of the following statements is FALSE?

(A) Infants normally get their first tooth at around 6 months of age.
(B) Premature eruption of the incisors can result in poor feeding.
(C) Acetaminophen is a good choice for treatment of teething discomfort.
(D) Teeth present at birth should always be pulled.
(E) Benzocaine gels can produce harmful side effects.

14-11. The cause of infant colic is

(A) a gastrointestinal abnormality
(B) a neurologic abnormality
(C) a psychological abnormality
(D) a nutritional abnormality
(E) unknown

14-12. The general definition of infant colic does NOT include

(A) crying during the day
(B) crying at least 3 h per day
(C) crying at least 3 days per week
(D) crying for at least 3 weeks
(E) crying that is inconsolable

14-13. The normal resting heart rate for a newborn is

(A) 75 to 115 bpm
(B) 85 to 125 bpm
(C) 110 to 150 bpm
(D) 140 to 200 bpm

14-14. The MOST common significant tachyarrhythmia in children is

(A) ventricular fibrillation (VF)
(B) ventricular tachycardia (VT)
(C) sinus tachycardia
(D) supraventricular tachycardia (SVT)

14-15. You are examining a patient with a suspected atrial septal defect (ASD). Select the physical examination or ECG finding that is NOT consistent with this diagnosis.

(A) a fixed-split second heart sound
(B) a holosystolic murmur
(C) a diastolic flow rumble at the lower left sternal border
(D) right ventricular hypertrophy

14-16. A 5-year-old male patient is examined and found to have a grade 3/6 systolic ejection murmur heard equally well at the left and right upper sternal borders with a systolic click. An ECG reveals mild left ventricular hypertrophy. The MOST likely diagnosis is

(A) ventricular septal defect
(B) atrial septal defect
(C) patent ductus arteriosus
(D) aortic stenosis
(E) pulmonic stenosis

14-17. A newborn patient is examined shortly after birth with a completely normal examination. At the 2-week examination a very faint systolic murmur is noted. The 2-month examination reveals a loud systolic murmur. The MOST likely diagnosis based on this information alone is

(A) ventricular septal defect
(B) atrial septal defect
(C) aortic stenosis
(D) pulmonic stenosis
(E) innocent heart murmur

14-18. Which of the following statements about pulmonic stenosis is TRUE?

(A) This condition affects more males than females.
(B) Patients do not require subacute bacterial precautions.
(C) ECG findings may include right axis deviation and right ventricular hypertrophy.
(D) A continuous machinery is audible at the upper left sternal border.

14-19. Which of the following symptoms suggests congestive heart failure in infants?

(A) diaphoresis with feedings
(B) fever
(C) cyanosis
(D) persistent irritability

14-20. A chest x-ray of a 1-year-old female patient reveals a prominent main pulmonary artery segment and normal pulmonary vascular markings. The MOST likely diagnosis is

(A) patent ductus arteriosus
(B) pulmonic stenosis
(C) aortic stenosis
(D) tetralogy of Fallot
(E) ventricular septal defect

14-21. Which of the following physical exam findings is suggestive of a heart defect?

(A) pectus excavatum
(B) a short, low-pitched systolic murmur
(C) fixed splitting of the second heart sound
(D) a continuous murmur heard at the upper left sternal border that is obliterated when the patient is supine

14-22. Which murmur description listed below is MOST consistent with a venous hum?

(A) a short, high-pitched systolic murmur heard maximally at the upper left sternal border
(B) a short, high-pitched murmur heard maximally above the clavicles on either side of the neck
(C) a continuous murmur that is heard at the upper left sternal border and is eliminated when the patient is supine
(D) a continuous murmur that is heard at the upper left sternal border and is persistent regardless of the patient's position

14-23. A 10-year-old patient reports to your office for a presports physical. Her history is unremarkable. Her cardiac auscultatory findings include a grade II/VI systolic ejection murmur that is high pitched and heard maximally at the upper left sternal border. No systolic click is audible. The MOST likely diagnosis is

(A) valvular pulmonic stenosis
(B) pulmonary flow murmur
(C) patent ductus arteriosus
(D) Still's murmur

14-24. Identify the TRUE statement regarding innocent heart murmurs from the list below.

(A) An innocent murmur is often pansystolic.
(B) Some diastolic murmurs can be considered innocent.
(C) All continuous murmurs are innocent.
(D) Ninety percent of all children will have an innocent heart murmur at some point.

14-25. The MOST reliable place to examine a patient for the presence of central cyanosis is the

(A) sclera
(B) oral mucosa
(C) nailbeds
(D) lips

14-26. Each of the following laboratory studies would be useful in assessing a patient with central cyanosis EXCEPT

(A) prothrombin time
(B) complete blood count
(C) arterial blood gas
(D) electrolyte levels

14-27. Which of the following neonates would be at risk for developing methemoglobinemia?

(A) an infant born at 35 weeks gestation (5 weeks premature)
(B) an infant who aspirated meconium during the delivery
(C) an infant born to a diabetic mother who took insulin during the pregnancy
(D) an infant who lives on a farm and is fed a powder formula

14-28. Which of the following is the CHARACTERISTIC antecedent of Reye's syndrome?

(A) viral infection
(B) bacterial infection
(C) fungal infection
(D) insect bite
(E) head trauma

14-29. Reye's syndrome may be precipitated by which of the following?

(A) aspirin
(B) acetaminophen
(C) dextromethorphan
(D) pseudoephedrine
(E) penicillin

14-30. In Reye's syndrome, damage to which of the following systems represents the GREATEST risk for serious sequelae for survivors?

(A) brain
(B) liver
(C) heart
(D) kidneys
(E) pancreas

14-31. A 4-year-old boy is brought to your office by his mother with complaints of overactivity and inattention. He has recently entered preschool and his mother is concerned that his behavior will result in problems at school when he gets older. She states that his behavior has been this way for about 2 months. She also states that her nephew has recently started on methylphenidate hydrochloride (Ritalin) and that it has helped his behavior. She asks you to prescribe Ritalin on a trial basis for her son. Which one of the following approaches would you recommend?

(A) 5 mg methylphenidate hydrochloride once a day for 1 month
(B) ask mother to complete the Conner's Parent Rating scale
(C) biofeedback techniques to help with monitoring overactivity
(D) do nothing now but schedule a follow-up appointment in 4 months
(E) a diet that eliminates preservatives and food coloring

14-32. All of the following statements about ADHD are TRUE EXCEPT

(A) The majority of children with ADHD demonstrate hyperactive and impulsive motor behavior.
(B) There is some evidence that children with ADHD demonstrate a greater incidence of neurologic "soft signs."
(C) Appropriate pharmacotherapy for ADHD has been shown to produce long-term benefit.
(D) Multimodal treatment strategies, including cognitive therapy and behavior management, are considered a desirable clinical approach.
(E) A diagnosis of ADHD is included in the Americans with Disabilities Act as a qualifying disability.

14-33. All of the following are considered criteria used to diagnose attention deficit hyperactivity disorder EXCEPT

(A) inattention
(B) hyperactivity
(C) long-term memory loss
(D) clinical impairment in social settings
(E) excessive talking

14-34. Medications used to treat attention deficit hyperactivity disorder include all of the following EXCEPT

(A) pemoline
(B) methylphenidate
(C) clonidine
(D) imipramine
(E) oxylate

14-35. The MOST common bacterial cause of osteomyelitis in children is

(A) *Escherichia coli*
(B) *Staphylococcus*
(C) *Haemophilus influenzae*
(D) group B *streptococcus*
(E) *Pseudomonas*

14-36. The MOST common age group for development of osteomyelitis in children is

(A) 1 to 2 years
(B) 2 to 4 years
(C) 6 to 14 years
(D) neonate
(E) 4 to 6 years

14-37. A 6-year-old male presents with palpable purpura present bilaterally over his shins. He also complains of knee and ankle pain. He had a URI prior to the onset of these symptoms. He is not on any medications. Platelet count and bleeding time are normal. The MOST likely diagnosis is

(A) immune thrombocytopenia purpura (ITP)
(B) Henoch-Schönlein purpura (HSP)
(C) hemophilia A
(D) infectious mononucleosis

14-38. A 9-year-old African-American child is brought to the energy room complaining of painful swelling in his hands and feet, as well as abdominal pain. He is feverish [39°C (102.2°F)] and tachycardiac (140 beats per minute). He has not been exposed to any known infectious diseases. His eyes appear icteric, and his liver is enlarged. Of the choices below, which is a likely diagnosis?

(A) sickle cell disease
(B) acute lymphocytic leukemia
(C) hemachromatosis
(D) Henoch-Schönlein purpura
(E) aplastic anemia

14-39. A 3-week-old infant is seen for persistent crying and anorexia. The baby has vomited four times in 24 h and passed no stools in 3 days. On exam, the infant appears dehydrated and has abdominal distention with loud bowel sounds. The MOST likely diagnosis is

(A) diverticulitis
(B) ulcerative colitis
(C) colonic polyposis
(D) cholecystolithiasis
(E) congenital Hirschsprung's disease

14-40. A 4-day-old infant is seen in your office with the complaint of excessive regurgitation and two large vomits in the last 2 days. On exam there is a mass effect right of the midline in the epigastric area. Which of the following is the MOST likely diagnosis?

(A) pyloric stenosis
(B) gastric carcinoma
(C) esophageal atresia
(D) peptic ulcer disease
(E) Zenker's diverticulum

14. PEDIATRICS

ANSWERS

14-1. **The correct answer is A.** Choice B is incorrect; this is not accomplished until age 4. Choice C is incorrect; this is not accomplished until age 5. Choice D is incorrect; this is not accomplished until after age 5. [Reichman J: Growth and development in infancy and early childhood, in Moser RL (ed): *Primary Care for Physician Assistants*. New York, McGraw-Hill, 1998, chap 15–6.]

14-2. **The correct answer is D.** Choice A is incorrect; children at this age are just beginning to speak and words are first appearing. Choice B is incorrect; at this age children have a limited vocabulary and speak in two-word phrases. Choice C is incorrect; at this age children have a moderate vocabulary and speak in very short (three-word) sentences; speech is not yet mature until age 4. [Reichman J: Growth and development in infancy and early childhood, in Moser RL (ed): *Primary Care for Physician Assistants*. New York, McGraw-Hill, 1998, chap 15–6.]

14-3. **The correct answer is B.** Choice A is incorrect because this milestone is generally accomplished by age 2. Choice C is incorrect because this milestone is generally accomplished by age 3. Choice D is incorrect because this milestone is generally accomplished by age 3 as well. [Reichman J: Growth and development in infancy and early childhood, in Moser RL (ed): *Primary Care for Physician Assistants*. New York, McGraw-Hill, 1998, chap 15–6.]

14-4. **The correct answer is D.** Choice A describes the rooting reflex. Choice B describes the palmar grasp. Choice C describes the Babinski response. [Reichman J: Growth and development in infancy and early childhood, in Moser RL (ed): *Primary Care for Physician Assistants*. New York, McGraw-Hill, 1998, chap 15–6.]

14-5. **The correct answer is B.** Choice A is incorrect; many children at age 2 cannot speak intelligibly 90 percent of the time. The rule of thumb is that children should speak intelligibly most of the time by age 3. Choice C is incorrect; stuttering at age 2 occurs as children are still learning to enunciate. Stuttering is not considered an indication for referral until age 5. [Reichman J: Growth and development in infancy and early childhood, in Moser RL (ed): *Primary Care for Physician Assistants*. New York, McGraw-Hill, 1998, chap 15–6.]

14-6. **The correct answer is D.** Total fat intake for children age 2 and older should constitute 30 percent or less of caloric intake, with saturated fats and polyunsaturated fats providing less than 10 percent each. Monounsaturated fats should provide 10 percent or more of caloric intake from fat. Most importantly, a well-balanced high-nutrition diet will teach good eating habits early. [Paterson KB: Pediatric nutrition, in Moser RL (ed): *Primary Care for Physician Assistants*. New York, McGraw-Hill, 1998, chap 15–1.]

14-7. **The correct answer is D.** Regular whole cow's milk is not suitable for infants since it can cause gastrointestinal bleeding and inappropriate renal load, although after 6 months, cow's milk can be used with a reasonable diet of solid foods. It must also be noted, however, that cow's milk is low in vitamin C and iron, which would need to be provided by the diet. Appropriate pediatric recommendations encourage the use of regular milk at a later age. [Paterson KB: Pediatric nutrition, in Moser RL (ed): *Primary Care for Physician Assistants*. New York, McGraw-Hill, 1998, chap 15–1.]

14-8. **The correct answer is C.** Premature infants are defined as those who are less than 270 days gestation and 2500 g (5.5 lb). Small-for-gestational-age infants are similar— although usually full term, they have some degree of intrauterine growth failure, low birth weights, and general growth retardation. Lengths of maternal labor are in no way related to an infant's premature status. [Paterson KB: Pediatric nutrition, in Moser RL (ed): *Primary Care for Physician Assistants*. New York, McGraw-Hill, 1998, chap 15–1.]

14-9. **The correct answer is B.** Fluoride content of human milk is generally low and a supplement administered through a dropper is recommended at about 2 weeks of age. Otherwise, a breast-fed infant should be monitored for iron, vitamin D, and protein intake. Vitamin K administered parenterally is needed, especially since infants consume a very small amount of milk during the first few hours of life. [Paterson KB: Pediatric nutrition, in Moser RL (ed): *Primary Care for Physician Assistants*. New York, McGraw-Hill, 1998, chap 15–1.]

14-10. **The correct answer is D.** Neonatal teeth need not be pulled, although this continues to be a common practice, with the belief that the teeth may dislodge and choke the infant. [Dehn R: Teething, in Moser RL (ed): *Primary Care for Physician Assistants*. New York, McGraw-Hill, 1998, chap 15–5.]

14-11. **The correct answer is E.** The cause of infant colic is unknown. Although theories abound, there is no common etiology. [Dehn R: Colic, in Moser RL (ed): *Primary Care for Physician Assistants*. New York, McGraw-Hill, 1998, chap 15–2.]

14-12. **The correct answer is A.** Crying during the day is not indicative of colic. Colic is more likely to occur in the evening hours. [Dehn R: Colic, in Moser RL (ed): *Primary Care for Physician Assistants*. New York, McGraw-Hill, 1998, chap 15–2.]

14-13. **The correct answer is C.** The normal resting heart rate of the newborn is 110 to 150 bpm. [Asprey DP: Pediatric arrhythmias, in Moser RL (ed): *Primary Care for Physician Assistants*. New York, McGraw-Hill, 1998, chap 15–9.]

14-14. **The correct answer is D.** SVT is the most common tachyarrhythmia. VF and VT are quite rare in children and sinus tachycardia is not a serious arrhythmia but rather a normal variation of sinus rhythm. [Asprey DP: Pediatric arrhythmias, in Moser RL (ed): *Primary Care for Physician Assistants*. New York, McGraw-Hill, 1998, chap 15–9.]

14-15. **The correct answer is B.** A holosystolic murmur is characteristic of a ventricular septal defect (VSD), not an ASD. The typical murmur associated with an ASD is an ejection murmur heard maximally in the pulmonic region. [Asprey DP: Congenital heart disease, in Moser RL (ed): *Primary Care for Physician Assistants*. New York, McGraw-Hill, 1998, chap 1–2.]

14-16. **The correct answer is D.** The presence of a click suggests valvular stenosis of either the aortic or pulmonic valve (given that mitral valve prolapse is not a choice). The presence of mild left ventricular hypertrophy (LVH) is indicative of aortic stenosis. [Asprey DP: Congenital heart disease, in Moser RL (ed): *Primary Care for Physician Assistants*. New York, McGraw-Hill, 1998, chap 1–2.]

14-17. **The correct answer is A.** Because the pulmonic pressure changes from systemic (equal to the left ventricle) to approximately one-fifth of systemic during the first 3 months of life, a VSD murmur becomes audible and then progressively louder as the pressure difference between the left and right ventricle becomes greater. [Asprey DP: Congenital heart disease, in Moser RL (ed): *Primary Care for Physician Assistants*. New York, McGraw-Hill, 1998, chap 1–2.]

14-18.   The correct answer is C.   Patients with significant pulmonic stenosis will have right axis deviation and RVH. [Asprey DP: Congenital heart disease, in Moser RL (ed): *Primary Care for Physician Assistants*. New York, McGraw-Hill, 1998, chap 1–2].

14-19.   The correct answer is A.   For infants, one of the most vigorous activities they do is to feed (either bottle or breast). Consequently, they will have diaphoresis during this mild form of exercise. [Asprey DP: Congenital heart disease, in Moser RL (ed): *Primary Care for Physician Assistants*. New York, McGraw-Hill, 1998, chap 1–2.]

14-20.   The correct answer is B.   Patients with pulmonic stenosis may have a dilated main pulmonary artery segment due to poststenotic dilation but will not have increased pulmonary vascular markings because there is no left-to-right shunting of blood. [Asprey DP: Congenital heart disease, in Moser RL (ed): *Primary Care for Physician Assistants*. New York, McGraw-Hill, 1998, chap 1–2.]

14-21.   The correct answer is C.   Fixed splitting of the second heart sound is an abnormal finding and usually occurs with an atrial septal defect. The other findings listed are normal findings. Pectus excavatum is not associated with congenital heart disease. [Asprey DP: Congenital heart disease, in Moser RL (ed): *Primary Care for Physician Assistants*. New York, McGraw-Hill, 1998, chap 1–2.]

14-22.   The correct answer is C.   The key to identifying the venous hum is that it is a continuous murmur that is typically obliterated or at least greatly reduced in intensity when the patient is supine. [Asprey DP: Pediatric innocent (functional) heart murmurs, in Moser RL (ed): *Primary Care for Physician Assistants*. New York, McGraw-Hill, 1998, chap 15–8.]

14-23.   The correct answer is B.   The absence of a click makes valvular pulmonic stenosis very unlikely. The patent ductus arteriosus murmur is continuous. A Still's murmur is usually heard at the lower left sternal border and is low pitched. [Asprey DP: Pediatric innocent (functional) heart murmurs, in Moser RL (ed): *Primary Care for Physician Assistants*. New York, McGraw-Hill, 1998, chap 15–8.]

14-24.   The correct answer is D.   Any murmur that is pansystolic or diastolic only should be considered pathologic. Some continuous murmurs, such as a patent ductus arteriosus, are not innocent. [Asprey DP: Pediatric innocent (functional) heart murmurs, in Moser RL (ed): *Primary Care for Physician Assistants*. New York, McGraw-Hill, 1998, chap 15–8.]

14-25.   The correct answer is B.   The oral mucosa is the most reliable anatomic location to examine for central cyanosis. The nailbeds and lips will often appear cyanotic in patients who have peripheral cyanosis but not necessarily central cyanosis. [Asprey DP: Neonatal cyanosis, in Moser RL (ed): *Primary Care for Physician Assistants*. New York, McGraw-Hill, 1998, chap 15–3.]

14-26.   The correct answer is A.   Prothrombin time is used to assess for the presence of deficiencies in the coagulation system of the blood. Each of the other tests is useful in assessing for possible etiologies of central cyanosis. [Asprey DP: Neonatal cyanosis, in Moser RL (ed): *Primary Care for Physician Assistants*. New York, McGraw-Hill, 1998, chap 15–3.]

14-27.   The correct answer is D.   An infant who lives on a farm and is fed powder formula is at great risk for developing methemeglobinemia. Methemeglobinemia is caused by ingestion of nitrates that may be present in untreated water systems such as individual-family wells. [Asprey DP: Neonatal cyanosis, in Moser RL (ed): *Primary Care for Physician Assistants*. New York, McGraw-Hill, 1998, chap 15–3.]

14-28. **The correct answer is A.** Reye's syndrome characteristically is preceded by a viral illness followed by vomiting and a progressive lethargy. It has an acute onset and is potentially fatal. It evolves to an encephalopathy that may be precipitated by salicylates administered during an episode of chickenpox or influenza. [Schymanski TJ: Reye's syndrome, in Moser RL (ed): *Primary Care for Physician Assistants*. New York, McGraw-Hill, 1998, chap 15–4.]

14-29. **The correct answer is A.** The salicylates, such as aspirin, that may be administered during an episode of chickenpox or influenza are thought to precipitate Reye's syndrome. Under what circumstances salicylates serve as a cofactor toxin in a susceptible child is still unknown. [Schymanski TJ: Reye's syndrome, in Moser RL (ed): *Primary Care for Physician Assistants*. New York, McGraw-Hill, 1998, chap 15–4.]

14-30. **The correct answer is A.** Although Reye's syndrome is a multisystem disease affecting the brain, heart, kidneys, liver, muscle tissue, and pancreas, damage to the brain tissue can have the most serious and yet underidentified sequelae. Among survivors, long-term follow-up will be of greatest importance for assisting the family in managing neurologic and psychological manifestations of learning and/or behavioral problems that can result in significant family stress. [Schymanski TJ: Reye's syndrome, in Moser RL (ed): *Primary Care for Physician Assistants*. New York, McGraw-Hill, 1998, chap 15–4.]

14-31. **The correct answer is B.** In 3- and 4-year-old children, overactivity and inattention are not necessarily indicators of later difficulties with attention deficit hyperactivity disorder (ADHD). Because of these normal developmental trends, a 12-month duration of symptoms should be observed for this age group, rather than the 6 months recommended in the DSM-IV for older children. The Conner's Parent Rating scale would, however, provide a baseline of observable behaviors that could be followed over time. [Naylor KE: Disruptive and negativistic behavior problems in children and adolescents, in Moser RL (ed): *Primary Care for Physician Assistants*. New York, McGraw-Hill, 1998, chap 15–7.]

14-32. **The correct answer is C.** Despite the often dramatic short-term effect that medication can have on the clinical symptoms of ADHD, there is still little evidence that the short-term benefits translate to an improved long-term prognosis for children. Multimodal treatment strategies are considered to be a desirable clinical approach to ADHD, which is thought to be a disability under ADA. [Naylor KE: Disruptive and negativistic behavior problems in children and adolescents, in Moser RL (ed): *Primary Care for Physician Assistants*. New York, McGraw-Hill, 1998, chap 15–7.]

14-33. **The correct answer is C.** According to the DSM-IV, the core clinical features of this disorder include impulsivity, distractibility, an inability to sustain attention and/or concentration, and developmentally inappropriate activity levels. Impairment from symptoms must be present in two or more settings. Long-term memory loss has not been associated with ADHD. [Naylor KE: Disruptive and negativistic behavior problems in children and adolescents, in Moser RL (ed): *Primary Care for Physician Assistants*. New York, McGraw-Hill, 1998, chap 15–7.]

14-34. **The correct answer is E.** Psychostimulants remain the most common treatment for ADHD. Approximately 70 percent of ADHD children treated with stimulants show significant improvement in attention, hyperactivity, and impulsivity. Stimulants include methylphenidate, dextroamphetamine, and pemoline. Tricyclic antidepressants, including imipramine, desipramine, and amitriptyline, are the most frequent alternatives. Clonidine, an antihypertensive compound, has also been found to be an effective treatment. [Naylor KE: Disruptive and negativistic behavior problems in children and adolescents, in Moser RL (ed): *Primary Care for Physician Assistants*. New York, McGraw-Hill, 1998, chap 15–7.]

14-35. The correct answer is B.   Most cases of acute hematogenous osteomyelitis in all age groups are caused by *Staphylococcus aureus. Haemophilus influenzae* and *Streptococcus* in children and infants, while important and problematic, are fewer in number than the more common *Staphylococcus.* [Cohen SM: Osteomyelitis, in Moser RL (ed): *Primary Care for Physician Assistants.* New York, McGraw-Hill, 1998, chap 10–17.]

14-36. The correct answer is C.   The 6 to14 age group has the highest incidence of osteomyelitis. It has been suggested that just prior to closure of the growth plates is the time of most turbulent blood flow in the area of the epiphysis. This has been theorized to increase seeding of hematogenous infection spread from distant sites such as nasopharynx. [Cohen SM: Osteomyelitis, in Moser RL (ed): *Primary Care for Physician Assistants.* New York, McGraw-Hill, 1998, chap 10–17.]

14-37. The correct answer is B.   HSP occurs most often in males at a median age of 6 years. It is a vasculitis whose most characteristic manifestation is a rash that often consists of purpura on the lower extremities. Arthralgias involving the knees and ankles are also a common manifestation. ITP would have a decreased platelet count. In hemophilia A, the bleeding time is prolonged. Infectious mononucleosis presents with a sore throat. [Deasy J: Henoch-Schönlein purpura, in Moser RL (ed): *Primary Care for Physician Assistants.* New York, McGraw-Hill, 1998, chap 8–7.]

14-38. The correct answer is A.   Children with sickle cell disease often present with painful swelling of the hands and feet, as well as pain in the abdomen and back. These children are often asymptomatic in early months of life. [Wrigley DS: Sickle cell anemia, in Moser RL (ed): *Primary Care for Physician Assistants.* New York, McGraw-Hill, 1998, chap 8–3.]

14-39. The correct answer is E.   Congenital Hirschsprung's causes constipation with eventual obstruction due to a small rectal vault and aganglionic colon. The other choices may mimic constipation but are not common in infants or toddlers. It is always important to recognize constipation as a symptom rather than a disease. As a symptom, constipation may herald a disease process but is not a disease in and of itself. [Heinly AP: Constipation, in Moser RL (ed): *Primary Care for Physician Assistants.* New York, McGraw-Hill, 1998, chap 6–6.]

14-40. The correct answer is A.   Nausea and vomiting are the presenting symptoms in infants with pyloric stenosis. There may be increased regurgitation because of the full stomach but a violent episode of vomiting will occur as the stomach attempts to empty itself. The mass is the stenotic sphincter. Esophageal atresia and Zenker's diverticulum are esophageal diseases that would present with regurgitation only and no mass effect. Adults can develop a similar process termed *gastric outlet syndrome* usually secondary to duodenal ulceration and subsequent scarring. [Heinly AP: Nausea and vomiting, in Moser RL (ed): *Primary Care for Physician Assistants.* New York, McGraw-Hill, 1998, chap 6–19.]

SECTION 15
PSYCHIATRY

15. PSYCHIATRY

QUESTIONS

DIRECTIONS: Each question below contains suggested responses. Choose the **one** **best** response to each question.

15-1. Treatment of eating disorders INITIAL focus is on

(A) individual psychotherapy
(B) normalization of the nutritional status
(C) hospitalization
(D) family psychotherapy
(E) treatment of depression

15-2. All of the following factors are related to a good prognosis for anorexia nervosa EXCEPT

(A) young age of onset
(B) supportive family
(C) lower educational achievement
(D) improvement in body image after weight gain
(E) good initial ego strength

15-3. Approximately what percent of anorexic patients are believed to have an associated major depressive syndrome?

(A) none
(B) 10 percent
(C) 50 percent
(D) 75 percent
(E) 100 percent

15-4. The motivation for attempted suicide (parasuicide or suicidal gesture) is likely to include all of the following EXCEPT

(A) a cry for help
(B) catharsis (to provide relief following a stressor)
(C) to create a change in a relationship
(D) response to a terminal illness
(E) to punish another individual

15-5. The MOST powerful predictor of suicide is

(A) past history of suicide attempt
(B) family history of suicide
(C) cluster A personality disorder
(D) female gender
(E) classic mania

15-6. Suicide is the most serious complication of depression and is seen in what percentage of depressed patients?

(A) 50 percent
(B) 25 percent
(C) 15 percent
(D) 10 percent
(E) 1 percent

15-7. The MOST crucial psychological factor predictive of suicide is

(A) poor problem-solving ability
(B) impulsive personality traits
(C) belief in religious prohibitions against suicide
(D) empathy toward survivors
(E) degree of hopelessness

15-8. The PRIMARY goals of suicide intervention include all of the following EXCEPT

(A) determine the patient's specific risk factors
(B) immediate hospitalization in a locked psychiatric unit
(C) protect the patient from himself or herself
(D) instill ethical/moral barriers to committing suicide
(E) remove the underlying distress

15-9. The psychiatric disorder conferring the GREATEST risk of suicide is

(A) depression
(B) schizophrenia
(C) borderline personality disorder
(D) mania
(E) panic disorder

15-10. Patients with generalized anxiety disorder (GAD) tend to seek treatment

(A) in psychiatric settings
(B) early in the course of the disorder
(C) for physical symptoms
(D) during acute anxiety attacks
(E) for secondary phobias

15-11. The MOST robust symptom of mania is

(A) increased goal-directed activity
(B) auditory hallucinations, which reflect underlying delusions
(C) increased sleep
(D) the patient has good insight into the development of symptoms

15-12. Being able to distinguish atypical mania from classic mania is important because

(A) they represent two different disease processes
(B) they may require a different treatment approach
(C) classic mania is much more difficult to treat
(D) patients with atypical mania are potentially more dangerous

15-13. In distinguishing schizophrenia from mania, the schizophrenic patient is more likely to exhibit

(A) disturbance of mood
(B) pressured speech
(C) mood-congruent delusions
(D) formal thought disorder

15-14. The MOST likely comorbid psychiatric disorder found in bipolar affective disorder patients is

(A) alcoholism
(B) attention deficit disorder
(C) schizophrenia
(D) delirium

15-15. Symptoms of lithium toxicity include

(A) tremor, nausea and vomiting, diarrhea, confusion
(B) elevated liver function studies
(C) parkinsonian symptoms, muscle stiffness, restlessness
(D) polyuria, increased thirst, drowsiness, tremor

15-16. The PRIMARY role of antipsychotics/neuroleptics in treating mania is

(A) induction of sleep
(B) mood stabilization
(C) treating flight of ideas, delusions, psychomotor agitation, and combativeness
(D) prevention of future manic episodes

15-17. Electroconvulsive therapy (ECT) should NOT be used under which situation?

(A) pregnancy
(B) severe cardiovascular disease
(C) while the patient is taking lithium
(D) in treatment of resistant patients

15-18. In the treatment of manic disorders, mood stabilizer therapy should be continued

(A) until the patient develops signs of toxicity
(B) until the manic episode ends and the patient develops good insight
(C) indefinitely
(D) at least 4 to 6 months after cessation of manic episode

15-19. Vegetative symptoms of depression include all of the following EXCEPT

(A) guilt, low self-esteem, and hopelessness
(B) initial, middle, and/or terminal insomnia
(C) psychomotor agitation or retardation
(D) fatigue and anergia
(E) anorexia or hyperphagia

15-20. Melancholic depression (often called endogenous depression) is characterized by

(A) the presence of delusions and/or hallucinations
(B) significant psychomotor symptoms, such as catatonia
(C) hypersomnia, hyperphagia, and rejection sensitivity
(D) terminal insomnia, anorexia, and excessive guilt
(E) presence or history of an expansive (manic or hypomanic) episode

15-21. When compared with patients with major depressive disorder, dysthymic patients tend to demonstrate

(A) more vegetative symptoms
(B) less fatigue and fewer social-motivational symptoms
(C) a more acute onset
(D) more persistence of symptoms
(E) less response to environmental stressors

15-22. Characteristics more likely to be found in depression secondary to another medical problem include all of the following EXCEPT

(A) absence of a family history of affective disorder
(B) greater cognitive impairment
(C) more severe initial episode
(D) poorer response to antidepressant therapy
(E) subclinical hypothyroidism

15-23. Predictors of a positive response to psychopharmacologic treatment of depression include all of the following EXCEPT

(A) psychotic symptoms
(B) vegetative symptoms
(C) family history of affective disorder
(D) acute onset
(E) history of positive response

15-24. The "gold standard" for treatment of depression is

(A) tricyclic antidepressants
(B) selective serotonin reuptake inhibitors
(C) lithium
(D) electroconvulsive therapy (ECT)
(E) monoamine oxidase inhibitors

15-25. Tyramine may precipitate a hypertensive crisis during pharmacotherapy with

(A) selective serotonin reuptake inhibitors
(B) bupropion
(C) monoamine oxidase inhibitors
(D) tricyclics or heterocyclics
(E) lithium

15-26. Children who are at risk for developing anxiety as adults often

(A) have paradoxical reactions to anxiolytics
(B) are behaviorally inhibited
(C) have depressive symptoms
(D) are hyperactive
(E) are quiet as infants

15-27. The principal feature of generalized anxiety disorder is

(A) perfectionist behavior
(B) self-denigrating cognitions
(C) worry out of proportion to the situation
(D) repeated anxiety attacks
(E) excessive fear in social situations

15-28. Buspirone may be helpful in treating

(A) specific phobias
(B) patients with prior history of benzodiazepine addiction
(C) benzodiazepine withdrawal
(D) panic disorder
(E) generalized anxiety disorder

15-29. The KEY characteristic of panic disorder is

(A) recurrent panic attacks with fear of recurrence
(B) agoraphobia seriously interfering with function
(C) irrational fear of evaluation by others
(D) recurrent attacks of hyperventilation
(E) rapid response to antidepressant therapy

15-30. The PRIMARY drugs used to treat obsessive-compulsive disorder (OCD)

(A) inhibit dopamine
(B) act as CNS stimulants
(C) increase norepinephrine activity
(D) have strong anxiolytic properties
(E) increase serotonin activity

15-31. Increased risk for developing posttraumatic stress disorder (PTSD) is associated with

(A) older age
(B) absence of psychiatric symptoms
(C) immediate debriefing
(D) use of physical force
(E) low physiologic response to the original trauma

15-32. The MOST common complications of panic disorder (PD) are

(A) depression and substance abuse
(B) benzodiazepine abuse and addiction
(C) suicide and homicide
(D) coronary artery disease and hypertension
(E) borderline and dependent personality disorders

15-33. Which of the following reflects the percentage of persons over 65 years of age who experience sleep disturbances?

(A) 20 percent
(B) 35 percent
(C) 50 percent
(D) 65 percent
(E) 80 percent

15-34. Which of the following age groups uses the largest percentage of prescribed sleep medications in the United States?

(A) 13- to 20-year-olds
(B) 21- to 30-year-olds
(C) 31- to 40-year-olds
(D) 41- to 50-year-olds
(E) over 50-year-olds

15-35. Which of the following is the MOST common cause of insomnia?

(A) depression
(B) anxiety
(C) sleep apnea
(D) alcohol use
(E) caffeine use

15. PSYCHIATRY

ANSWERS

15-1. **The correct answer is B.** Normalization of the nutritional status, particularly in patients with severe symptoms of malnutrition, is always the first focus of treatment of eating disorders. [Davison M: Eating disorders: Anorexia and bulimia, in Moser RL (ed): *Primary Care for Physician Assistants*. New York, McGraw-Hill, 1998, chap 16–1.]

15-2. **The correct answer is C.** High educational achievement has been found to be associated with a better prognosis for anorexia nervosa. [Davison M: Eating disorders: Anorexia and bulimia, in Moser RL (ed): *Primary Care for Physician Assistants*. New York, McGraw-Hill, 1998, chap 16–1.]

15-3. **The correct answer is C.** Half of all patients with anorexia nervosa are believed to have an associated major depressive syndrome. [Davison M: Eating disorders: Anorexia and bulimia, in Moser RL (ed): *Primary Care for Physician Assistants*. New York, McGraw-Hill, 1998, chap 16–1.]

15-4. **The correct answer is D.** The motivation of parasuicide is usually interpersonal. The typical attempter is young, female, impulsive, takes few precautions to be discovered, has low suicidal preoccupation and intent, and uses a "soft" method, such as overdose or cutting. This is in contrast to the typical completer who is older, male, isolated, depressed, takes many precautions to avoid discovery, plans the suicide, has high suicidal preoccupation and intent, uses "harder" methods, and is more likely to be self-directed in motivation. [St. John D: Suicide, in Moser RL (ed): *Primary Care for Physician Assistants*. New York, McGraw-Hill, 1998, chap 16–7.]

15-5. **The correct answer is A.** A past history of suicide attempt is found in 30 to 40 percent of completers and 10 to 15 percent of attempters will eventually complete a suicide. While 11 percent of suicide victims have a family history of suicide, it is a weak predictor. Patients with cluster B personality disorders have a higher risk of both attempts and completions. Suicide is rare in patients with cluster C personality disorders. Risk of completion is higher (4:1) among men than women. Patients with mixed mania are at higher risk of committing suicide, and this seems to be related to the degree of depression present. [St. John D: Suicide, in Moser RL (ed): *Primary Care for Physician Assistants*. New York, McGraw-Hill, 1998, chap 16–7.]

15-6. **The correct answer is C.** Fifteen percent of depressed patients will ultimately complete a suicide. Depression is the most treatable risk factor for suicide. Risk is especially high shortly after discharge from inpatient psychiatric treatment, perhaps because patients tend to be discharged before all symptoms have responded to antidepressant therapy. The patient remains hopeless but has developed the resolve and energy to complete a suicide. [St. John D: Suicide, in Moser RL (ed): *Primary Care for Physician Assistants*. New York, McGraw-Hill, 1998, chap 16–7.]

15-7.   **The correct answer is E.**   The degree of hopelessness cues the clinician to the patient's desperation. Poor problem-solving abilities, impulsivity and aggressiveness, dichotomous thinking, cognitive rigidity, a poor concept of future, negative self-concept, and a sense of isolation are associated cognitive disorders. Empathy toward survivors is a protective factor, as are religious prohibitions. [St. John D: Suicide, in Moser RL (ed): *Primary Care for Physician Assistants.* New York, McGraw-Hill, 1998, chap 16–7.]

15-8.   **The correct answer is B.**   Most patients with suicidal ideation will not require inpatient treatment. Many are ambivalent and even frightened by their suicidal thoughts and respond to an empathic, supportive, and nonjudgmental approach, utilizing a cognitive style of therapy. Indications for inpatient treatment include the need to shelter the patient from harm, create a protective support system, examine the patient in an undrugged state, observe the patient to determine risk, remove the patient from a stressful situation, stabilize the patient's emotional state, and reassess outpatient treatment. [St. John D: Suicide, in Moser RL (ed): *Primary Care for Physician Assistants.* New York, McGraw-Hill, 1998, chap 16–7.]

15-9.   **The correct answer is A.**   Fifteen percent of patients with depression will complete a suicide, which is 5 to 7 times that of the general population. Ten percent of schizophrenics will commit suicide, often during a relatively nonpsychotic period. While patients with borderline personality disorder are not at increased risk, they tend to make suicidal gestures and engage in self-harm behaviors much more commonly. Manic patients appear to be at increased risk in the mixed state, and the risk appears to be dependent on the degree of depression present. Patients with panic disorder are at slightly increased risk. [St. John D: Suicide, in Moser RL (ed): *Primary Care for Physician Assistants.* New York, McGraw-Hill, 1998, chap 16–7.]

15-10.   **The correct answer is C.**   Patients with GAD tend to seek treatment for physical symptoms. They present to primary care practitioners and present to psychiatrists usually only by referral. They tend to present late, often years after the onset of symptoms. Phobias rarely present for treatment. [St. John D: Anxiety and panic disorders, in Moser RL (ed): *Primary Care for Physician Assistants.* New York, McGraw-Hill, 1998, chap 16–3.]

15-11.   **The correct answer is A.**   Auditory hallucinations are found only in psychotic mania, occurring in 20 to 50 percent of acutely manic patients. Decreased need for sleep characterizes mania. Increasing sleep is a therapeutic goal. Patients usually demonstrate very poor insight. [St. John D: Manic disorders, in Moser RL (ed): *Primary Care for Physician Assistants.* New York, McGraw-Hill, 1998, chap 16–6.]

15-12.   **The correct answer is B.**   Lithium is the mood stabilizer of choice for classic mania, while valproate/divalproex and carbamazepine are the mood stabilizers of choice for atypical manias. These are variants of the same disease process. Classic mania is usually easier to treat, though both forms may be difficult. Dangerousness is associated with irritable mood and paranoia. [St. John D: Manic disorders, in Moser RL (ed): *Primary Care for Physician Assistants.* New York, McGraw-Hill, 1998, chap 16–6.]

15-13.   **The correct answer is D.**   Formal thought disorder is a distinguishing symptom of schizophrenia. Disturbance of mood is a hallmark of affective disorders. Mania is an affective disorder. Schizophrenia is a thought disorder. Unusual forms of speech, demonstrating the underlying thought disorder, are more typical of schizophrenia. Schizophrenic delusions are usually detached from mood. [St. John D: Manic disorders, in Moser RL (ed): *Primary Care for Physician Assistants.* New York, McGraw-Hill, 1998, chap 16–6.]

15-14.   **The correct answer is A.**   Alcoholism is found in 34 to 50 percent of patients with bipolar affective disorders. Attention deficit disorder is to be differentiated from mania and is not found at a higher rate in manic patients. Schizophrenia is not found at a higher rate in manic patients. Delirium is to be differentiated from mania. [St. John D: Manic disorders, in Moser RL (ed): *Primary Care for Physician Assistants.* New York, McGraw-Hill, 1998, chap 16–6.]

15-15. **The correct answer is A.** Benign elevation of liver function tests may be found with use of valproate/divalproex and carbamazepine, but is not evidence of toxicity. Parkinsonian symptoms, muscle stiffness, and restlessness are side effects of neuroleptics. Polyuria, increased thirst, drowsiness, and tremor are common side effects of lithium, but do not indicate potential toxicity. [St. John D: Manic disorders, in Moser RL (ed): *Primary Care for Physician Assistants.* New York, McGraw-Hill, 1998, chap 16–6.]

15-16. **The correct answer is C.** Benzodiazepines are most effective for inducing sleep. The mood stabilizers currently used are lithium, valproate/divalproex, and carbamazepine. As a rule, neuroleptics should be discontinued once the manic episode is controlled. Patients with affective disorders may be at higher risk for the development of tardive dyskinesia. [St. John D: Manic disorders, in Moser RL (ed): *Primary Care for Physician Assistants.* New York, McGraw-Hill, 1998, chap 16–6.]

15-17. **The correct answer is C.** Concurrent use of lithium and electroconvulsive therapy may put the patient at higher risk of organic brain syndrome. Choices A, B, and C are indications to use electroconvulsive therapy in treating acute manic states. [St. John D: Manic disorders, in Moser RL (ed): *Primary Care for Physician Assistants.* New York, McGraw-Hill, 1998, chap 16–6.]

15-18. **The correct answer is D.** After 4 to 6 months, the mood stabilizer that controlled the manic symptoms may be gradually tapered. Signs of toxicity indicate the need to decrease the dose, which may occur as a manic patient on lithium stabilizes. Discontinuation of mood stabilizer therapy, even when secondary causes of mania have been controlled, may lead to a recurrence of mania. Each recurrence increases treatment resistance. Indefinite use of mood stabilizers should be considered after three manic episodes, especially in atypical mania. [St. John D: Manic disorders, in Moser RL (ed): *Primary Care for Physician Assistants.* New York, McGraw-Hill, 1998, chap 16–6.]

15-19. **The correct answer is A.** Vegetative symptoms of depression include changes in sleep, psychomotor activity, physical energy, appetite, concentration, and even constipation. Diurnal variation of symptoms are also considered a vegetative symptom. Guilt, low self-esteem, and hopelessness result from negative cognitions relating to the past, present, and future, and are cognitive symptoms of depression. Affective symptoms represent the basic abnormality in depression and include depressed mood, dysphoria, anhedonia, irritability, paranoia, brooding, crying, and anxiety. [St. John D: Depression, in Moser RL (ed): *Primary Care for Physician Assistants.* New York, McGraw-Hill, 1998, chap 16–5.]

15-20. **The correct answer is D.** Melancholic depression is characterized by terminal insomnia (early morning awakening), anorexia and weight loss, excessive guilt, psychomotor retardation or agitation, and a diurnal variation where the symptoms are worse in the morning and improve throughout the day. The presence of delusions or hallucinations characterizes psychotic depression. Catatonia, mutism, peculiar movements, and/or excessive purposeless motor activity are seen in catatonic depression. Atypical features tend to be the opposite of melancholia and include hyperphagia with weight gain, hypersomnia, leaden paralysis, and rejection sensitivity. The presence of expansive mood symptoms characterizes bipolar variants. [St. John D: Depression, in Moser RL (ed): *Primary Care for Physician Assistants.* New York, McGraw-Hill, 1998, chap 16–5.]

15-21. **The correct answer is D.** Dysthymic patients tend to have fewer vegetative symptoms, and more fatigue, social-motivational, and cognitive symptoms. Dysthymia tends to have a more insidious onset, be more unrelenting, and is characterized more by anger, irritability, self-pity, and reactivity to environmental stressors. Persistence of symptoms is the most discriminating factor in making a diagnosis of dysthymia. [St. John D: Depression, in Moser RL (ed): *Primary Care for Physician Assistants.* New York, McGraw-Hill, 1998, chap 16–5.]

15-22. The correct answer is E. The absence of a family history of affective disorders, greater cognitive impairment, a more severe initial episode, and poorer response to antidepressant therapy are more characteristic features of depression that occurs secondary to another primary medical disorder than of primary depression. Subclinical hypothyroidism (elevated TSH with normal T3 and T4, or blunted TSH response to administration of thyrotropin-releasing hormone) is more common in patients with affective disorders, but is unrelated to secondary depression. [St. John D: Depression, in Moser RL (ed): *Primary Care for Physician Assistants.* New York, McGraw-Hill, 1998, chap 16–5.]

15-23. The correct answer is A. Predictors of a good response to psychopharmacotherapy are associated with vegetative symptoms, hypersomnia, melancholia, acute onset, absence of family dysfunction, history of prior response, and family history of mood disorder. Patients with psychotic symptoms are more difficult to treat, usually requiring the addition of a neuroleptic and often requiring longer prophylaxis. [St. John D: Depression, in Moser RL (ed): *Primary Care for Physician Assistants.* New York, McGraw-Hill, 1998, chap 16–5.]

15-24. The correct answer is D. The "gold standard" for treatment is ECT, which is effective in 80 percent of depressed patients, and even works in acutely manic patients. All other antidepressants are equally effective, although certain classes and agents may be more effective for specific types of depression and under special circumstances. Lithium may be used as a primary treatment modality, though its less tolerable side-effect profile usually relegates it to a secondary or augmentation status. [St. John D: Depression, in Moser RL (ed): *Primary Care for Physician Assistants.* New York, McGraw-Hill, 1998, chap 16–5.]

15-25. The correct answer is C. A hypertensive crisis may occur when a patient taking (or having recently discontinued) a nonreversible monoamine oxidase (MAO) inhibitor ingests tyramine. There are no special dietary or drug precautions to take with the other common antidepressants. Reversible MAO inhibitors, which may not present the risk of a hypertensive crisis, are being tested, but are not currently available in the United States. Selective MAO inhibitors (e.g., selegiline, which is currently indicated for treating Parkinson's disease) may also be associated with this risk, especially at higher doses. [St. John D: Depression, in Moser RL (ed): *Primary Care for Physician Assistants.* New York, McGraw-Hill, 1998, chap 16–5.]

15-26. The correct answer is B. Children at risk for the development of anxiety disorders display behavioral inhibition, separation anxiety, and school phobia. They tend to be irritable as infants, shy and fearful as toddlers, and quiet and cautious as school children. Depression frequently develops secondary to anxiety disorders in adulthood. [St. John D: Anxiety and panic disorders, in Moser RL (ed): *Primary Care for Physician Assistants.* New York, McGraw-Hill, 1998, chap 16–3.]

15-27. The correct answer is C. Worry out of proportion to the situation is the principal feature of generalized anxiety disorder (GAD). Anxiety tends to be diffuse and ongoing, not episodic, in GAD. Perfectionistic behaviors may characterize obsessive-compulsive personality disorder. Self-denigrating cognitions are more characteristic of depressive disorders. Fear in social situations is more characteristic of social phobia. [St. John D: Anxiety and panic disorders, in Moser RL (ed): *Primary Care for Physician Assistants.* New York, McGraw-Hill, 1998, chap 16–3.]

15-28. The correct answer is E. Buspirone can be used to treat general anxiety symptoms, such as those found in GAD, as well as to augment antidepressants. It is not effective in treating panic attacks. Buspirone cannot be substituted for benzodiazepines (BZDs), will not treat BZD withdrawal symptoms, and tends not to be effective in patients with histories of BZD addiction. Specific phobias do not respond to psychopharmacology. [St. John D: Anxiety and panic disorders, in Moser RL (ed): *Primary Care for Physician Assistants.* New York, McGraw-Hill, 1998, chap 16–3.]

15-29.   The correct answer is A.   Recurrent panic attacks with fear of recurrence are the key characteristics of panic disorder. Agoraphobia, fear of being in a place or situation where escape may be difficult, may develop in some, but not all, patients with panic disorder, and may even occur in the absence of panic disorder. Irrational fear of evaluation by others is found in patients with social phobia. Hyperventilation is one of many symptoms of panic disorder. Many panic-disorder patients notice an increase in anxiety symptoms when antidepressant therapy is initiated, as they tend to be very sensitive to medication side effects. [St. John D: Anxiety and panic disorders, in Moser RL (ed): *Primary Care for Physician Assistants*. New York, McGraw-Hill, 1998, chap 16–3.]

15-30.   The correct answer is E.   Psychopharmacology of OCD utilizes drugs that increase serotonin activity, which include clomipramine and selective serotonin reuptake inhibitors (e.g., fluoxetine, fluvoxamine, paroxetine, sertraline). Antidepressants with primarily noradrenergic, dopaminergic, CNS stimulant, or anxiolytic effects have no primary role in treating OCD, though they may be useful as augmenting agents for individual patients. [St. John D: Anxiety and panic disorders, in Moser RL (ed): *Primary Care for Physician Assistants*. New York, McGraw-Hill, 1998, chap 16–3.]

15-31.   The correct answer is D.   Increased risk for the development of PTSD symptoms is associated with the use of physical force, display of a weapon, physical injury, young age, poor preparation (e.g., military), prior abuse history, and the presence of psychiatric symptoms prior to the event. Immediate and thorough debriefing is thought to decrease the risk of developing disabling PTSD following a severe stressor. The intensity of the physiologic response to the event appears to be the most significant predictor of outcome and course. [St. John D: Anxiety and panic disorders, in Moser RL (ed): *Primary Care for Physician Assistants*. New York, McGraw-Hill, 1998, chap 16–3.]

15-32.   The correct answer is A.   Depression and substance abuse are the most common complications of panic disorder. BZD abuse and addiction are uncommon in patients treated for PD. In fact, patients tend to fear addiction and are commonly undertreated. The suicide rate is somewhat higher in PD, but homicide risk is not increased. Patients with PD are at higher risk of mortality secondary to CAD, and hypertension is more common in patients with PD, but it is unclear if they are complications, comorbid, or part of the disease process. Panic attacks and anxiety may be present in patients with personality disorders, which are usually present prior to the onset of PD. [St. John D: Anxiety and panic disorders, in Moser RL (ed): *Primary Care for Physician Assistants*. New York, McGraw-Hill, 1998, chap 16–3.]

15-33.   The correct answer is C.   More than half of all elderly persons over age 65 and living at home suffer from sleep disturbances. An estimated two-thirds of those living in assisted living facilities also complain of chronic insomnia. Nighttime insomnia with daytime sleepiness can be a product of normal aging, a primary sleep disorder, medical illness, or the result of an adverse reaction to a medication. [Mosier WA: Sleep disorders, in Moser RL (ed): *Primary Care for Physician Assistants*. New York, McGraw-Hill, 1998, chap 16–2.]

15-34.   The correct answer is E.   Although the percentage of people over 50 years old only accounts for 25 percent of the total US population, they are prescribed over 50 percent of all sleep medications. The majority of their sleep disorders involve a combination of psychological and organic factors. [Mosier WA: Sleep disorders, in Moser RL (ed): *Primary Care for Physician Assistants*. New York, McGraw-Hill, 1998, chap 16–2.]

15-35.   The correct answer is A.   Mood disorders, such as depression, are the most prevalent underlying causes of insomnia. Depression affects all stages of sleep. Careful medical, psychiatric, and drug histories are necessary to uncover the principle cause of insomnia in each individual patient. [Mosier WA: Sleep disorders, in Moser RL (ed): *Primary Care for Physician Assistants*. New York, McGraw-Hill, 1998, chap 16–2.]

SECTION 16
RESPIRATORY

16. RESPIRATORY

QUESTIONS

DIRECTIONS: Each question below contains suggested responses. Choose the **one best** response to each question.

16-1. Acute bronchitis is MOST commonly caused by

(A) enteric pathogens
(B) viruses
(C) bacteria aspirated from nasopharynx
(D) inhalation of bacteria
(E) fungal elements

16-2. Pathogens that MOST often cause acute bronchitis include all of the following EXCEPT

(A) adenovirus, corona virus, and influenza A and B
(B) *Haemophilus influenzae, Mycoplasma pneumoniae,* and *Moraxella catarrhalis*
(C) *Streptococcus pneumoniae, Staphylococcus aureus,* and pneumococcus
(D) *Klebsiella pneumoniae, Legionella pneumophila,* and *Bacteriodes fragilis*
(E) rhinovirus, parainfluenza, and respiratory syncytial virus

16-3. The PRIMARY risk factor(s) for emphysema or chronic bronchitis is/are

(A) environmental or occupational dust
(B) air pollution and second-hand smoke
(C) cigarette smoke
(D) alpha$_1$-antitrypsin deficiency
(E) respiratory problems (i.e., viral illness, asthma) as a child

16-4. In emphysema, the disease process is characterized by

(A) mucous plugging of small airways
(B) inflammation
(C) smooth-muscle hypertrophy
(D) destruction of alveolar walls
(E) edema

16-5. The INITIAL treatment for COPD is

(A) methylxanthines (theophylline)
(B) corticosteroids (prednisone)
(C) bronchodilators
(D) cromolyn sodium (Intal)
(E) supplemental oxygen therapy

16-6. Patients with COPD should be vaccinated against

(A) hepatitis B
(B) pneumonia and influenza
(C) mumps, measles, rubella
(D) *Haemophilus influenzae* (Hib)
(E) tetanus, diphtheria

16-7. The HIGHEST incidence of COPD in Americans is in which ethnic group?

(A) Hispanic-Americans
(B) Native Americans
(C) Asian-Americans
(D) Caucasians
(E) African-Americans

16-8. The MOST prominent physical finding(s) in COPD is/are

(A) low position of diaphragm by percussion
(B) jugular venous distention
(C) diminished breath sounds and coarse rhonchi
(D) pedal edema
(E) prolonged expiration

16-9. Which of the following would be the MOST useful when attempting to determine if a patient is suffering from coal worker's pneumoconiosis, asbestosis, or silicosis?

(A) documented occupational history
(B) chest x-ray findings
(C) pulmonary function test abnormalities
(D) physical examination findings

16-10. What are the FIRST visible signs on a chest x-ray in an individual with asbestosis?

(A) pleural plaques
(B) honeycombed lungs
(C) progressive massive fibrosis
(D) small, round parenchymal opacities

16-11. Which of the following medications induces bronchodilatation via its anticholinergic effects on the muscarinic receptors of the bronchial smooth muscle?

(A) pirbuterol
(B) ipratropium bromide
(C) theophylline
(D) albuterol

16-12. A patient with bronchiectasis presents with fever, cough, and purulent sputum production. The MOST likely diagnosis and course of treatment is

(A) diagnosis: chronic exacerbation
     treatment: continue present treatment plan
(B) diagnosis: worsening of disease
     treatment: order pulmonary function test and
     prescribe bronchodilators
(C) diagnosis: infection
     treatment: order chest x-ray and prescribe
     antibiotics
(D) diagnosis: viral illness
     treatment: wait and see
(E) diagnosis: infection
     treatment: prescribe empiric antibiotics and
     order sputum culture/sensitivity

16-13. The MOST frequently diagnosed AIDS-defining illness is

(A) cytamegaloviris (CMV)
(B) Kaposi's sarcoma
(C) *Pneumocystis carinii* pneumonia (PCP)
(D) pneumococcus
(E) toxoplasmosis

16-14. Which of the following blood gas abnormalities is common in PCP?

(A) hypocapnia
(B) increased oxygen-diffusing capacity
(C) reduced carbon dioxide–diffusing capacity
(D) respiratory acidosis
(E) none of the above

16-15. Mild to moderate PCP in a patient with no prior history and no other medical conditions should be treated with

(A) atovaquone
(B) clindamycin
(C) dapsone
(D) pentamidine
(E) trimethoprim/sulfamethoxazole

16-16. The MOST serious side effect of PCP treatment is

(A) diarrhea
(B) hemolysis
(C) neutropenia
(D) rash
(E) renal failure

16-17. Which of the following is the MOST common debilitating disease occurring among persons of European Caucasian descent?

(A) cystic fibrosis
(B) multiple sclerosis
(C) muscular dystrophy
(D) poliomyelitis
(E) diabetes mellitus

16-18. Which of the following confirms the diagnosis of cystic fibrosis?

(A) sweat test
(B) x-ray
(C) blood test
(D) ultrasound
(E) CT scan

16-19. The MOST common cause of pleural trauma is

(A) infection
(B) noxious agents
(C) rib fractures
(D) collagen and vascular disease
(E) neoplastic problems

16-20. Which physical sign is MOST pathognomonic of pleurisy?

(A) temperature greater than 38.3°C (101° F)
(B) nausea and vomiting
(C) a pleural friction rub
(D) an elevated white blood count
(E) an elevated sedimentation rate

16-21. The MOST common cause of community-acquired pneumonia (CAP) is

(A) *Mycoplasma pneumoniae*
(B) *Klebsiella pneumoniae*
(C) *Streptococcus pneumoniae*
(D) *Haemophilus influenzae*

16-22. A 45-year-old, previously healthy female presents with the sudden onset of chills, fever, a cough productive of rust-colored sputum, and pleuritic chest pain. She is a nonsmoker and a nondrinker. Auscultation of the chest reveals crackles in the right lower lobe. Of the following, the MOST appropriate INITIAL diagnostic test would be

(A) sputum culture
(B) complete blood count (CBC)
(C) urine antigen test for pneumococcus
(D) chest x-ray

16-23. The MOST likely diagnosis for the patient in the previous question is

(A) *Mycoplasma* pneumonia
(B) pneumococcal pneumonia
(C) staphylococcal pneumonia
(D) pneumonia caused by *Klebsiella pneumoniae*

16-24. The drug of choice for treating pneumonia caused by *Legionella pneumophila* is

(A) penicillin
(B) a second-generation cephalosporin
(C) erythromycin
(D) amoxicillin

16-25. A 23-year-old female who lives in a college dormitory develops a sore throat followed by a non-productive cough that lingers. During the course of her illness she did experience a low-grade fever. The MOST likely diagnosis is

(A) *Mycoplasma* pneumonia
(B) pneumococcal pneumonia
(C) staphylococcal pneumonia
(D) *Legionella* pneumonia
(E) pneumonia caused by *Klebsiella pneumoniae*

16-26. A 65-year-old male with COPD is diagnosed with pneumonia. Based on his clinical presentation, he is going to be treated as an outpatient. He has no medication allergies. The BEST antibiotic choice for empirical treatment would be (according to American Thoracic Society Guidelines)

(A) erythromycin
(B) cefuroxine axetil (Ceftin) (second-generation cephalosporin)
(C) tetracycline
(D) penicillin

16-27. Which of the following radiographic studies in a stable patient would help elicit a small pneumothorax?

(A) AP chest x-ray
(B) lateral chest x-ray
(C) lateral oblique chest x-ray
(D) end-inspiration chest x-ray
(E) PA chest x-ray

16-28. You are called to the intensive care unit to see a 45-year-old patient on a ventilator who has suddenly developed severe dyspnea, tachypnea, tachycardia, jugular venous distention, extreme agitation, asymmetric chest expansion, tracheal deviation, poor oxygen saturation, and signs of cyanosis. An hour earlier the resident replaced the Swan-Ganz catheter via a left subclavian approach without incident. The patient's blood pressure is 60/40, CVP is 14, venous saturation is 78%. The MOST likely diagnosis in the above-stated scenario is

(A) right-sided hemopneumothorax
(B) left-sided tension pneumothorax
(C) iatrogenic right-sided pneumothorax
(D) pulmonary embolus
(E) improper ventilator settings

16-29. The classical triad of hemoptysis, pleuritic chest pain, and dyspnea

(A) is a common manifestation of pulmonary embolism
(B) occurs most commonly with large pulmonary emboli
(C) shows large filling defects on VQ scans
(D) likely represents peripherally located emboli
(E) is a contraindication for anticoagulant therapy

16-30. Chest x-ray findings in pulmonary embolus

(A) do not manifest themselves for 12 to 24 h
(B) are manifested primarily as Kerley B lines
(C) reveal flattened diaphragms
(D) are of little value after the first 8 h
(E) reveal multiple radiolucent areas

16. RESPIRATORY

ANSWERS

16-1. **The correct answer is B.** Viruses are the most common cause of acute bronchitis. The others can cause bronchitis but are not the most common. [O'Hara MM: Acute bronchitis in previously healthy individuals, in Moser RL (ed): *Primary Care for Physician Assistants.* New York, McGraw-Hill, 1998, chap 17–2.]

16-2. **The correct answer is D.** These bacterial pathogens are not usually seen in acute bronchitis in previously healthy individuals, but may be seen in those who have some reason for immunocompromise. Viruses are the primary cause of infection in acute bronchitis. [O'Hara MM: Acute bronchitis in previously healthy individuals, in Moser RL (ed): *Primary Care for Physician Assistants.* New York, McGraw-Hill, 1998, chap 17–2.]

16-3. **The correct answer is C.** The other answers can cause COPD without smoking and are considered secondary causes. It has been documented that cigarette smoke will increase the decline of pulmonary function. [O'Hara MM: Chronic obstructive pulmonary disease: Emphysema and chronic bronchitis, in Moser RL (ed): *Primary Care for Physician Assistants.* New York, McGraw-Hill, 1998, chap 17–11.]

16-4. **The correct answer is D.** The mechanism of the destruction of the alveolar walls is theorized to be an imbalance between the proteases that cause the breakdown of elastin in the alveolar walls and the enzymes responsible for the repair of elastin. The other answers describe the process involved in chronic bronchitis. [O'Hara MM: Chronic obstructive pulmonary disease: Emphysema and chronic bronchitis, in Moser RL (ed): *Primary Care for Physician Assistants.* New York, McGraw-Hill, 1998, chap 17–11.]

16-5. **The correct answer is C.** Bronchodilators are used to reverse bronchospasm of small airways. Theophylline and corticosteroids are adjuncts to treatment. Cromolyn is an anti-inflammatory agent that is used in the treatment of asthma. Oxygen is used when the $PaCO_2$ drops below 55 mm Hg. [O'Hara MM: Chronic obstructive pulmonary disease: Emphysema and chronic bronchitis, in Moser RL (ed): *Primary Care for Physician Assistants.* New York, McGraw-Hill, 1998, chap 17–11.]

16-6. **The correct answer is B.** The patients should have pneumonia and flu vaccinations because of the potential to cause bronchospasm and scarring of lung tissue. Hib is a childhood vaccination. An MMR booster is recommended between ages 21 and 40, regardless of pulmonary status. Tetanus/diphtheria is recommended every 10 years, regardless of pulmonary status. [O'Hara MM: Chronic obstructive pulmonary disease: Emphysema and chronic bronchitis, in Moser RL (ed): *Primary Care for Physician Assistants.* New York, McGraw-Hill, 1998, chap 17–11.]

16-7. **The correct answer is D.** Currently the highest incidence is among Caucasian males. The rate is increasing in other groups as more women and teenagers take up smoking. [O'Hara MM: Chronic obstructive pulmonary disease: Emphysema and chronic bronchitis, in Moser RL (ed): *Primary Care for Physician Assistants.* New York, McGraw-Hill, 1998, chap 17–11.]

16-8. **The correct answer is E.** Due to narrowing of the airways, patients will have prolonged expirations that may be evident as they speak. The other findings are usually seen in more severe disease. [O'Hara MM: Chronic obstructive pulmonary disease: Emphysema and chronic bronchitis, in Moser RL (ed): *Primary Care for Physician Assistants.* New York, McGraw-Hill, 1998, chap 17–11.]

16-9. **The correct answer is A.** Although chest x-ray and pulmonary function test results could make you more suspicious for one over the other, the findings on these tests are very similar for all three. The type of dust the patient is exposed to is the most accurate method to determine the pathogen. [Scott PM: Occupational pneumoconiosis, in Moser RL (ed): *Primary Care for Physician Assistants.* New York: McGraw-Hill, 1998. chap 17–10.]

16-10. **The correct answer is D.** Progressive massive fibrosis and pleural plaques are both seen in the later stages of asbestosis, not as the first visible signs. Honeycombed lungs are generally associated with silicosis. [Scott PM: Occupational pneumoconiosis, in Moser RL (ed): *Primary Care for Physician Assistants.* New York, McGraw-Hill, 1998, chap 17–10.]

16-11. **The correct answer is B.** Pirbuterol and albuterol are both beta-agonists and exert their effects on the beta receptors, not the muscarinic. Theophylline affects the smooth muscles and pulmonary blood vessels via an unknown mechanism. [Scott PM: Occupational pheumonconiosis, in Moser RL (ed): *Primary Care for Physician Assistants.* New York, McGraw-Hill, 1998, chap 17–10.]

16-12. **The correct answer is E.** Fever and purulent sputum production indicate infection. Patients with bronchiectasis often have unusual pathogens. It is important to determine the pathogen to direct appropriate antibiotic therapy. [Heymann CJ: Bronchiectasis, in Moser RL (ed): *Primary Care for Physician Assistants.* New York, McGraw-Hill, 1998, chap 17–3.]

16-13. **The correct answer is C.** Despite advances in diagnosis, treatment, and prophylaxis, PCP remains the most frequently encountered respiratory illness in HIV with nearly 20,000 new cases reported to the CDC annually. [O'Connell CB: *Pneumocystis carinii* pneumonia, in Moser RL (ed): *Primary Care for Physician Assistants.* New York, McGraw-Hill, 1998, chap 17–6.]

16-14. **The correct answer is C.** A reduction in the carbon dioxide–diffusing capacity is almost universal in PCP. If the reduction is not seen on arterial blood gas analysis, the likelihood of PCP is very low. Other abnormalities include hypoxemia and respiratory alkalosis. [O'Connell CB: *Pneumocystis carinii* pneumonia, in Moser RL (ed): *Primary Care for Physician Assistants.* New York, McGraw-Hill, 1998, chap 17–6.]

16-15. **The correct answer is E.** TMP/SMX is the drug of choice in PCP. It is given orally in any patient with mild to moderate disease who is able to tolerate oral medication. The other choices represent alternative therapies for people not able to tolerate TMP/SMX. [O'Connell CB: *Pneumocystis carinii* pneumonia, in Moser RL (ed): *Primary Care for Physician Assistants.* New York, McGraw-Hill, 1998, chap 17–6.]

16-16. **The correct answer is C.** TMP/SMX is the most frequently used drug against PCP. It may cause a rash, fever, abnormal liver enzymes, or, most seriously, neutropenia. Pentamidine is associated with renal failure as well as neutropenia and other side effects. Other anti-PCP regimens are also associated with neutropenia, fever, hemolysis, and other side effects. By far the most serious consequence of the therapy is neutropenia. Patients must be monitored closely. [O'Connell CB: *Pneumocystis carinii* pneumonia, in Moser RL (ed): *Primary Care for Physician Assistants.* New York, McGraw-Hill, 1998, chap 17–6.]

16-17. **The correct answer is A.** Cystic fibrosis (CF) is the most common genetic disease among individuals with European Caucasian heritage. The incidence is approximately 1 in 2500 live births. There are an estimated 30,000 Americans afflicted with the disease. It is additionally estimated that over 8 million Americans are symptom-free carriers of the CF gene. [Mosier WA: Cystic fibrosis (muscoviscidosis), in Moser RL (ed): *Primary Care for Physician Assistants*. New York, McGraw-Hill, 1998, chap 7–1.]

16-18. **The correct answer is A.** To confirm the diagnosis of cystic fibrosis a sweat test, utilizing pilocarpine iontophoresis, is performed. Sweat chloride concentrations exceeding 60 meq/L are found in 98 percent of all patients with CF. 60 meq/L confirms the diagnosis for patients under 20 years of age. 80 meq/L confirms the diagnosis for patients 20 years old and older. [Mosier WA: Cystic fibrosis (muscoviscidosis), in Moser RL (ed): *Primary Care for Physician Assistants*. New York, McGraw-Hill, 1998, chap 7–1.]

16-19. **The correct answer is C.** Rib fractures are the most common cause of pleural trauma. Infectious and noxious agents, and collagen, vascular, and neoplastic problems are not traumatic injuries. [Trudeau R: Pleurisy, in Moser RL (ed): *Primary Care for Physician Assistants*. New York, McGraw-Hill, 1998, chap 17–9.]

16-20. **The correct answer is C.** An elevated white blood count would be associated with infection; elevated sedimentation rate would be associated with inflammatory disease. Temperature, nausea, and vomiting are very nonspecific findings and could be related to many different pathologies. [Trudeau R: Pleurisy, in Moser RL (ed): *Primary Care for Physician Assistants*. New York, McGraw-Hill, 1998, chap 17–9.]

16-21. **The correct answer is C.** Studies show that 30 percent to 70 percent of community-acquired pneumonias are due to *Streptococcus pneumoniae*. [Deasy J: Pneumonia, in Moser RL (ed): *Primary Care for Physician Assistants*. New York, McGraw-Hill, 1998, chap 17–7.]

16-22. **The correct answer is D.** This patient presents with symptoms and signs typical of pneumococcal pneumonia. The presence of an infiltrate on the chest x-ray will confirm the diagnosis of pneumonia and should be the first test ordered. Once an infiltrate is documented on the chest x-ray, other tests can be done. [Deasy J: Pneumonia, in Moser RL (ed): *Primary Care for Physician Assistants*. New York, McGraw-Hill, 1998, chap 17–7.]

16-23. **The correct answer is B.** These clinical symptoms and signs are very typical of pneumococcal pneumonia. Mycoplasma usually has a gradual onset with nonproductive cough. Both staphylococcal pneumonia and pneumonia due to *Klebsiella pneumoniae* usually occur in debilitated persons or persons with a risk factor. [Deasy J: Pneumonia, in Moser RL (ed): *Primary Care for Physician Assistants*. New York, McGraw-Hill, 1998, chap 17–7.]

16-24. **The correct answer is C.** Erythromycin is the drug of choice. *Legionella* frequently produces beta-lactamase, so penicillins and cephalosporins usually are not effective. [Deasy J: Pneumonia, in Moser RL (ed): *Primary Care for Physician Assistants*. New York, McGraw-Hill, 1998, chap 17–7.]

16-25. **The correct answer is A.** Mycoplasma is most common in the younger age group and presents with a gradual onset and dry cough, often associated with pharyngitis. [Deasy J: Pneumonia, in Moser RL (ed): *Primary Care for Physician Assistants*. New York, McGraw-Hill, 1998, chap 17–7.]

16-26. **The correct answer is B.** A second-generation cephalosporin will provide coverage for *Streptococcus pneumoniae, Moraxella catarrhalis,* and *Haemophilus influenzae,* three common pathogens in the older age group with a comorbidity, such as COPD. [Deasy J: Pneumonia, in Moser RL (ed): *Primary Care for Physician Assistants*. New York, McGraw-Hill, 1998, chap 17–7.]

16-27. **The correct answer is D.**   The standard views without inspiration may miss a small pneumothorax. [Cassidy BA: Pneumothorax, in Moser RL (ed): *Primary Care for Physician Assistants*. New York, McGraw-Hill, 1998, chap 17–5.]

16-28. **The correct answer is B.**   This patient has a serious left-sided pneumothorax and needs immediate emergency management. [Cassidy BA: Pneumothorax, in Moser RL (ed): *Primary Care for Physician Assistants*. New York, McGraw-Hill, 1998, chap 17–5.]

16-29. **The correct answer is D.**   Happening in less than 20 percent of all patients with pulmonary embolism (PE), the classic symptoms tend to occur when the PE is located in the very periphery of the pulmonary arteries where the mortality rate is the lowest. [Cassidy BA: Pulmonary embolus, in Moser RL (ed): *Primary Care for Physician Assistants*. New York, McGraw-Hill, 1998, chap 17–8.]

16-30. **The correct answer is A.**   The evaluation of suspected PE should be multidisciplinary in nature. One pitfall, germane to the primary practitioner, is that radiographic changes may take 12 to 24 h to manifest and may therefore not show on the initial chest x-ray. [Cassidy BA: Pulmonary embolus, in Moser RL (ed): *Primary Care for Physician Assistants*. New York, McGraw-Hill, 1998, chap 17–8.]

SECTION 17
UROLOGY

17. UROLOGY

QUESTIONS

DIRECTIONS: Each question below contains suggested responses. Choose the **one best** response to each question.

17-1. Which is the MOST common reason that adult women develop urinary tract infections (UTIs)?

(A) improper wiping techniques after toileting
(B) not urinating often enough (holding it too long)
(C) sexual activity
(D) tampon use
(E) use of diaphragms

17-2. The MOST common reason that adult men over 40 develop urinary tract infections is

(A) exposure to sexually transmitted organisms
(B) a change in the pH of the urine that occurs with maturity
(C) excessive alcohol and sedentary lifestyle
(D) reduced resistance to bacterial microorganisms
(E) prostatic hypertrophy

17-3. Of all the organisms that can cause a urinary tract infection, MOST originate from

(A) the bloodstream
(B) the genital tract
(C) the intestinal tract
(D) the skin

17-4. Which of the following organisms is/are LEAST likely to cause a UTI?

(A) *Streptococcus* spp.
(B) *Enterobacter* spp.
(C) *Klebsiella* spp.
(D) *Escherichia coli*
(E) *Staphylococcus* spp.

17-5. Which chemical marker on a urine dipstick is MOST likely to be correlated with an infection?

(A) pH above 8.0
(B) positive nitrites
(C) specific gravity <1.000
(D) positive ketones
(E) positive monocytes

17-6. MATCHING: The color of the urine on gross examination can often give you a diagnostic clue. Match the following urine characteristics to a possible cause in the choices below.

(A) caused by methylene dye in the drug Urised
(B) caused by diabetes mellitus
(C) caused by intense hyperemia and bleeding
(D) caused by Pyridium
(E) caused by bacteriuria from enteric organisms in the urinary tract

____ fluorescent orange urine
____ red or pink urine
____ green or bluish urine
____ dark yellow, turbid, foul-smelling urine

17-7. Most women with classic UTI symptoms actually have a UTI. What do the others have in most cases? In other words, which one is your MOST likely differential diagnosis for the classic UTI?

(A) acute abdomen
(B) pelvic inflammatory disease (PID)
(C) vaginitis
(D) gastroenteritis
(E) menstrual cramps

17-8. In *infants*, urinary tract infections are more common in

(A) infant boys (under age 1)
(B) infant girls (under age 1)

17-9. Your 3-year-old patient with a confirmed UTI is allergic to sulfa. Which of the following medications would be a good second choice?

(A) Gantrisin
(B) Bactrim/Septra
(C) doxycycline
(D) amoxicillin
(E) Pediazole

17-10. Of the choices below, which would be the BEST for a first-trimester pregnant woman with a simple urinary tract infection?

(A) trimethoprim/sulfamethoxazole
(B) nitrofurantoin
(C) doxycycline
(D) tetracycline

17-11. Which of the urinary microorganisms is/are associated with renal lithiasis?

(A) *Proteus* spp.
(B) *Escherichia coli*
(C) *Pseudomonas* spp.
(D) *Staphylococcus saprophyticus*
(E) *Klebsiella* spp.

17-12. The BEST test for determining inflammation of the prostate is

(A) prostatic secretion culture
(B) >10 WBC/hpf in the prostatic secretions
(C) urine microscopic examination
(D) urine culture
(E) prostate-specific antigen

17-13. Which would be the BEST of the following therapy choices for acute prostatitis?

(A) trimethoprim/sulfamethoxazole (Bactrim/Septra) DS bid
(B) doxycycline (Vibramycin) 100 mg bid
(C) terazosin (Hytrin) starting with 1 mg HS, and increasing up to 10 mg
(D) ciprofloxacin (Cipro) 200 mg IV every 12 h
(E) ampicillin 1 gram IV every 6 h

17-14. Prostate-specific antigen is elevated in

(A) acute bacterial prostatitis
(B) chronic bacterial prostatitis
(C) chronic nonbacterial prostatitis
(D) prostatodynia
(E) bladder cancer

17-15. Which of the following is NOT a sign or symptom of acute prostatitis?

(A) fever
(B) tender prostate
(C) brownish-yellow-colored urine
(D) inability to urinate
(E) back pain

17-16. An afebrile 20-year-old male with pain during urination would MOST likely have

(A) acute bacterial prostatitis
(B) chronic bacterial prostatitis
(C) chronic nonbacterial prostatitis
(D) prostate cancer
(E) epididymitis

17-17. A sexually active 27-year-old heterosexual male presents with urethral symptoms and pain consistent with epididymitis. The most likely infectious agent is

(A) *Escherichia coli*
(B) *Chlamydia trachomatis*
(C) *Mycobacterium tuberculosis*
(D) *Neisseria gonorrhoeae*
(E) *Treponema pallidum*

17-18. In a 12-year-old male with symptoms of epididymitis, the MOST common differential diagnosis that must be ruled out quickly is

(A) acute orchitis
(B) congenital hydrocele
(C) spermatocele
(D) testicular torsion
(E) testicular tumor

17-19. In a homosexual male with acute epididymitis, the MOST likely causative organism would be

(A) *Chlamydia trachomatis*
(B) *Escherichia coli*
(C) *Haemophilus influenzae*
(D) *Neisseria gonorrhoeae*
(E) *Treponema pallidum*

17-20. A 65-year-old male with chronic prostatitis presents with epididymitis. The MOST likely causative microorganism is

(A) *Bacteroides fragilis*
(B) *Chlamydia trachomatis*
(C) *Escherichia coli*
(D) *Neisseria gonorrhoeae*
(E) *Treponema pallidum*

17-21. The complications of mumps orchitis include all the following EXCEPT

(A) testicular atrophy
(B) myocardial infarction
(C) sterility
(D) pulmonary infarction
(E) priapism

17-22. Which of the following is the LEAST likely to present with only 12 to 24 h of nausea and vomiting?

(A) otitis media
(B) renal failure
(C) pregnancy
(D) cellulitis
(E) acute gastroenteritis (AGE)

17-23. The glomerular filtration rate (GFR) that defines renal failure is

(A) <75% of normal
(B) <60% of normal
(C) <40% of normal
(D) <25% of normal
(E) <10% of normal

17-24. Of the following, the MOST sensitive test to differentiate prerenal from intrinsic (renal) types of acute renal failure is

(A) the urinary sodium index
(B) the urine specific gravity
(C) the urine osmolality
(D) the fractional excretion of sodium (FENa)
(E) the plasma BUN level at presentation

17-25. Of the following parameters, which would provide the LEAST information in determining the cause of a patient's acute renal failure?

(A) a 24-h urinary output
(B) a urine specific gravity
(C) a plasma BUN and creatinine value
(D) a urinary osmolality
(E) a urinary sodium value

17. UROLOGY

ANSWERS

17-1. **The correct answer is C.** Sexual activity increases the incidence of UTIs fiftyfold. Improper toileting habits are often blamed for children's infections, but this is not thought to be true in adult females. Tampon use has no correlation to UTIs, but an improperly fitting diaphragm may restrict the free flow of urine and contribute to a urinary tract infection. [Moser RL: Urinary tract infections, in Moser RL (ed): *Primary Care for Physician Assistants.* New York, McGraw-Hill, 1998, chap 18–6.]

17-2. **The correct answer is E.** Prostatic hypertrophy is the most common structural anomaly that results in urinary tract infection in men over 40. There is no change in urinary pH that is characteristic with maturity. The elderly male may have a reduced resistance to infection, but this does not occur as early as age 40. [Moser RL: Urinary tract infections, in Moser RL (ed): *Primary Care for Physician Assistants.* New York, McGraw-Hill, 1998, chap 18–6.]

17-3. **The correct answer is C.** Enteric organisms are the most frequent pathogens. Skin contaminants such as *Staphylococcus aureus* can result in urinary tract problems, but this is less common than intestinal tract organisms. [Moser RL: Urinary tract infections, in Moser RL (ed): *Primary Care for Physician Assistants.* New York, McGraw-Hill, 1998, chap 18–6.]

17-4. **The correct answer is A.** The enteric organisms (B, C, and D) are the most likely culprits, followed by *Staphylococcus.* Although *Streptococcus* is responsible for a small percentage of UTIs, it is the least likely from the list above. [Moser RL: Urinary tract infections, in Moser RL (ed): *Primary Care for Physician Assistants.* New York, McGraw-Hill, 1998, chap 18–6.]

17-5. **The correct answer is B.** Positive nitrites are a presumptive indicator of urinary tract infection on the chemical dipstick. [Moser RL: Urinary tract infections, in Moser RL (ed): *Primary Care for Physician Assistants.* New York, McGraw-Hill, 1998, chap 18–6.]

17-6. **The correct answer is D.** Pyridium is a fluorescent orange dye used for urinary tract discomfort. Often hoarded by patients from previous UTIs, it can often be seen in acute urine specimens.

The correct answer is C. UTIs are often accompanied by hematuria, which can tint the urine to bloodlike red, or pinkish.

The correct answer is A. Urised, used for urinary tract discomfort, characteristically will change the urine color to a green or greenish-blue color.

The correct answer is E. Dark yellow, turbid, or foul-smelling urine is common in acute infections. This is due in part to concentration and bacterial contaminants. [Moser RL: Urinary tract infections, in Moser RL (ed): *Primary Care for Physician Assistants.* New York, McGraw-Hill, 1998, chap 18–6.]

17-7. **The correct answer is C.** Up to 50 percent of UTI-symptomatic women who do not have a UTI, based on urinalysis or culture, have a vaginal infection of some sort, which can range from moniliasis to bacterial vaginosis. [Moser RL: Urinary tract infections, in Moser RL (ed): *Primary Care for Physician Assistants*. New York, McGraw-Hill, 1998, chap 18–6.]

17-8. **The correct answer is A.** Due to congenital urinary tract anomalies, infant boys have a higher rate of UTIs than infant girls. However, after age 1, the incidence is considerably higher in females. [Moser RL: Urinary tract infections, in Moser RL (ed): *Primary Care for Physician Assistants*. New York, McGraw-Hill, 1998, chap 18–6.]

17-9. **The correct answer is D.** Amoxicillin is a good choice for treating a simple UTI in a 3-year-old. It is effective and has a good compliance rate. All other medications contain sulfa, with the exception of doxycycline, which is contraindicated at that age. [Moser RL: Urinary tract infections, in Moser RL (ed): *Primary Care for Physician Assistants*. New York, McGraw-Hill, 1998, chap 18–6.]

17-10. **The correct answer is B.** Of the choices offered, nitrofurantoin is the best choice. Tetracycline-containing or related drugs are contraindicated, as is trimethoprim/sulfamethoxazole. [Moser RL: Urinary tract infections, in Moser RL (ed): *Primary Care for Physician Assistants*. New York, McGraw-Hill, 1998, chap 18–6.]

17-11. **The correct answer is A.** *Proteus* spp. are often associated with renal lithiasis. [O'Brien-Norton M: Renal lithiasis and pyelonephritis, in Moser RL (ed): *Primary Care for Physician Assistants*. New York, McGraw-Hill, 1998, chap 18–5.]

17-12. **The correct answer is B.** The presence of a significant number of leukocytes is more indicative of an infection or inflammation. [Dehn R: Prostatitis, in Moser RL (ed): *Primary Care for Physician Assistants*. New York, McGraw-Hill, 1998, chap 18–3.]

17-13. **The correct answer is D.** Although trimethoprim/sulfamethoxazole and doxycycline are frequently used, ciprofloxacin would be a better choice. [Dehn R: Prostatitis, in Moser RL (ed): *Primary Care for Physician Assistants*. New York, McGraw-Hill, 1998, chap 18–3.]

17-14. **The correct answer is A.** Acute infections of the prostate can cause elevations in the prostate-specific antigen, whereas chronic involvement is less likely to cause elevations. Prostatodynia is pain. Bladder cancer does not result in an elevation of the PSA level unless there is metastatic involvement. [Dehn R: Prostatitis, in Moser RL (ed): *Primary Care for Physician Assistants*. New York, McGraw-Hill, 1998, chap 18–3.]

17-15. **The correct answer is C.** Brownish-yellow-colored urine is not indicative of prostatitis, but is a common finding in hepatitis. Fever, tenderness, dysuria, and back pain are common complaints. [Dehn R: Prostatitis, in Moser RL (ed): *Primary Care for Physician Assistants*. New York, McGraw-Hill, 1998, chap 18–3.]

17-16. **The correct answer is C.** An afebrile 20-year-old is more likely to have a chronic nonbacterial prostatitis. Prostate cancer is highly unlikely in this age group. [Dehn R: Prostatitis, in Moser RL (ed): *Primary Care for Physician Assistants*. New York, McGraw-Hill, 1998, chap 18–3.]

17-17. **The correct answer is B.** Up to 70 percent of epididymitis in heterosexual males under the age of 35 is due to *Chlamydia trachomatis*. *Escherichia coli* is frequently the etiology in infants and children less than 5 years old, in homosexual males, and in men older than 35 years of age. *Neisseria gonorrhoeae* is a less common bacterial etiology in heterosexual males under the age of 35. *Mycobacterium tuberculosis* and *Treponema pallidum* are seen in chronic cases and/or in immunocompromised patients. [Riggs AR: Epididymitis/orchitis, in Moser RL (ed): *Primary Care for Physician Assistants*. New York, McGraw-Hill, 1998, chap 18–4.]

17-18. **The correct answer is D.** Testicular torsion, which deprives the testicle of blood flow, needs to be diagnosed and treated within 4 to 6 h to save the testicle. Acute orchitis, congenital hydrocele, and spermatocele typically are not problems that threaten the viability of the testis. Testicular tumor, although potentially fatal, is a condition that allows more time for evaluation. [Riggs AR: Epididymitis/orchitis, in Moser RL (ed): *Primary Care for Physician Assistants*. New York, McGraw-Hill, 1998, chap 18–4.]

17-19. **The correct answer is B.** In homosexual males performing unprotected anogenital intercourse, the most common cause of epididymitis is a coliform bacterium such as *E. coli*. *Haemophilus influenzae* has been isolated in one case. *C. trachomatis* and *N. gonorrhoeae* are typically seen in heterosexually acquired epididymitis. *T. pallidum* is usually a cause of chronic epididymitis. [Riggs AR: Epididymitis/orchitis, in Moser RL (ed): *Primary Care for Physician Assistants*. New York, McGraw-Hill, 1998, chap 18–4.]

17-20. **The correct answer is C.** *E. coli* causes 80 percent of prostate infections and commonly causes epididymitis in men over 35 with prostate problems. *B. fragilis* is an anaerobe that usually does not cause prostate infection unless there has been a transrectal prostate biopsy. *C. trachomatis, N. gonorrhoeae,* and *T. pallidum* are sexually acquired infections and are usually seen in epididymitis in males under the age of 35. [Riggs AR: Epididymitis/orchitis, in Moser RL (ed): *Primary Care for Physician Assistants*. New York, McGraw-Hill, 1998, chap 18–4.]

17-21. **The correct answer is B.** Myocardial infarction is not known to be a complication. The other complications are reported. [Riggs AR: Epidiymitis/orchitis, in Moser RL (ed): *Primary Care for Physician Assistants*. New York, McGraw-Hill, 1998, chap 18–4.]

17-22. **The correct answer is B.** If the patient exhibits transient nausea and vomiting, defined as lasting hours to a few days, look for acute etiologies. For nausea and/or vomiting lasting longer than a few days, consider chronic etiologies such as obstruction (complete or partial), carcinoma, brain tumor, and liver or renal failure, to name a few. [Sefcik DJ: Acute renal failure, in Moser RL (ed): *Primary Care for Physician Assistants*. New York, McGraw-Hill, 1998, chap 18–1.]

17-23. **The correct answer is E.** A GFR less than 10 percent of normal defines renal failure. GFR values less than 40 to 50 percent of normal are known as renal impairment. GFR values less than 20 to 39 percent of normal are discussed as renal insufficiency. [Sefcik DJ: Acute renal failure, in Moser RL (ed): *Primary Care for Physician Assistants*. New York, McGraw-Hill, 1998, chap 18–1.]

17-24. **The correct answer is D.** Although the other renal failure indices may offer some guidance as to the type of acute renal failure, the FENa is considered to be the most sensitive of the choices provided. [Sefcik DJ: Acute renal failure, in Moser RL (ed): *Primary Care for Physician Assistants*. New York, McGraw-Hill, 1998, chap 18–1.]

17-25. **The correct answer is A.** Since ARF is the result of numerous etiologies and may present as oliguric or nonoliguric, the knowledge of a 24-h urine output will offer limited assistance in determining the etiology of ARF. The other answers, however, provide information as renal failure indices and may offer help in differentiating prerenal from intrinsic (renal) ARF. [Sefcik DJ: Acute renal failure, in Moser RL (ed): *Primary Care for Physician Assistants*. New York, McGraw-Hill, 1998, chap 18–1.]

BIBLIOGRAPHY

Andreoli TE: *Cecil Essentials of Medicine*, 4th ed. Philadelphia, Saunders, 1997.

Fauci A, Braunwald E, Isselbacher KJ, et al (eds): *Harrison's Principles of Internal Medicine*, 14th ed. New York, McGraw-Hill, 1998.

Kelly WN, DuPont HL (eds): *Textbook of Internal Medicine*, 3d ed. Philadelphia, Lippincott-Raven, 1997.

Moser RL (ed): *Primary Care for Physician Assistants*. New York, McGraw-Hill, 1998.

ISBN 0-07-052406-8

90000